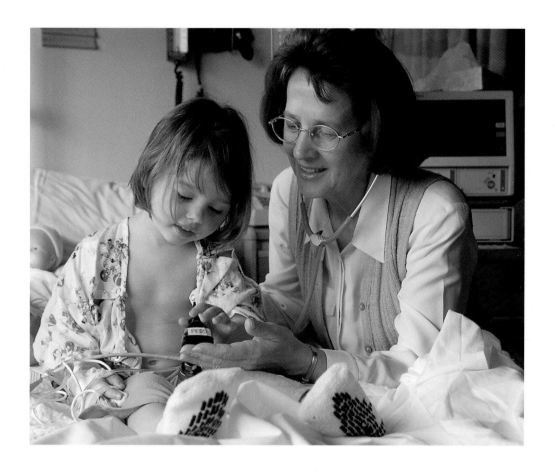

Being a Pediatrician

Text and Photography by
Travis Cavens, MD, FAAP
(Fellow of the American Academy of Pediatrics)

Published by Lake Publishing Company
2938 Laurel Road
Longview, WA 98632

COVER PHOTO: Dr. Phyllis Cavens with 4-year-old Madelynn Martin
TABLE OF CONTENTS PHOTO: Dr. Phyllis Cavens with Julie Garcia and her baby, Andrew

Library of Congress Catalog Card Number: 00-90053
Cavens, Travis R., 1935
Being a Pediatrician / text and photography by Travis R. Cavens
ISBN 0-9659385-2-2
1. Pediatrician 2. Cavens, Dr. Phyllis 3. American Academy of Pediatrics

Printed in Korea

Acknowledgements

The author is grateful to his wife, Phyllis, who is the inspiration for this book; to his daughter, Sonja, who, as a nurse in obstetrics, arranged many of the pictures; and to his son, Derek, who offered helpful advice in photography and who, along with David Rorden, edited the manuscript. He is also thankful to the staff of the Child and Adolescent Clinic; Dr. Cindy Cristofani of Legacy Emanuel Children's Hospital; Dr. Joel Alpert, past president of the American Academy of Pediatrics; Sherry Llewellyn of the AAP; Dr. Milton Arnold and Eve Black of the AAP California District IX Chapter; and the staff of St. John Medical Center in Longview, Washington.

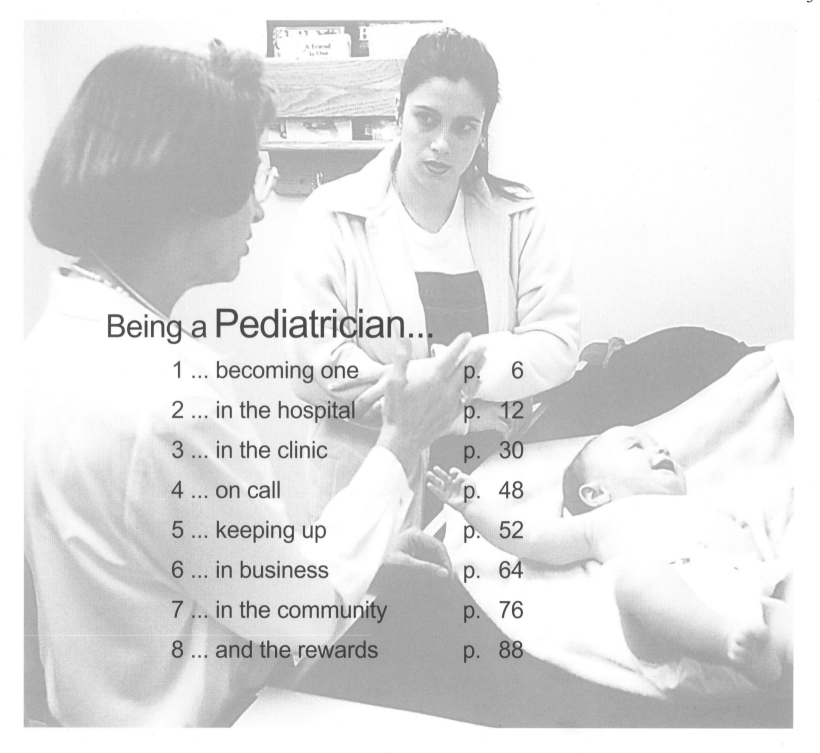

Being a Pediatrician...

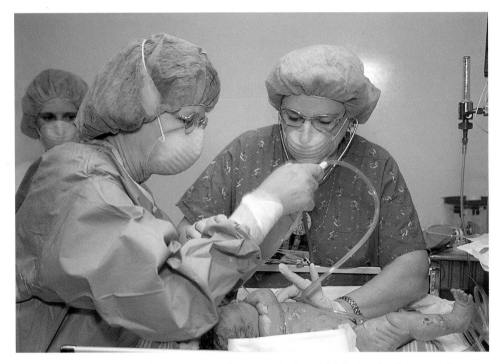

Pediatrician Dr. Phyllis Cavens cares for a new baby girl, Marley Anderson, who was just delivered by Caesarean section. A neonatal nurse, Sandi Nolden, monitors the baby's heart rate while an operating room nurse, Sonja Cavens, waits for blood samples.

Why this book

My high school dream of being a writer and photographer was resurrected recently when I laid aside my stethoscope and ototscope (the defining instruments of a pediatrician) and retired. My wife, Phyllis, however, is still immersed in the daily practice of pediatrics.

It dawned on me that I had a unique opportunity to create an insider's book about being a pediatrician, catching the joys, frustrations, and rewards of this blessed profession. I could follow my wife with notepad and camera as she left the quiet of our home each day to enter the hurly-burly of clinic and hospital practice.

I'm very proud of the pediatric profession. Even though its practitioners experience the same stresses that all doctors feel, pediatricians have a higher level of career satisfaction and a lower rate of suicide than any of the other medical specialties. The reason? They help children.

It is indeed a profession of joy, helping little ones bloom into young adults, full of life and promise. Instead of dealing with aging and dying generations, pediatricians work in an atmosphere of ongoing creation. Their job is not only to defy disease, but to guide the decades-long unfolding of new lives.

My doctor-wife, who is a very good pediatrician, does this very well, but she is not unique. She is representative, rather, of some 55,000 pediatricians in this country who open their exam room doors each morning and cheerfully greet their little friends with, "Hi there. I'm Dr. ...."

So, to all those pediatricians like her, I dedicate this book.

Travis Cavens, MD, FAAP

1 ... becoming one

Please Meet Phyllis Cavens

Dr. Phyllis Cavens is a general pediatrician whose two-acre home site is nestled in the midst of tall Douglas firs, trees that threaten to deplete the lawn below them as they cast their brooding, Pacific Northwest shadows.

In the 1920s, trees like those towering firs lured a Kansas City timber company to the state of Washington to build the world's largest lumber mill, creating at the same time a carefully planned city named Longview. The city, now with a population of 30,000, is spread out along the banks of the Columbia River.

I am Dr. Phyllis's husband and a fellow pediatrician. We moved to Longview in 1971 with our two small children, Derek and Sonja. In 1980, our town was hindered economically by the volcanic explosion of Mount St. Helens some 40 miles away, and so it has grown slowly. It still takes only 10 minutes for Phyllis to drive to her workplace, the Child and Adolescent Clinic.

With maturity and experience, Dr. Phyllis has reached the pinnacle of being a physician. Like pediatricians everywhere, she delights in the frequent encounters in the grocery store or church with her patients, little children whose eyes light up when they spot "my doctor."

The Child and Adolescent Clinic in Longview, a medical home for children of Southwest Washington.

In addition, Phyllis is a mother, wife, steelhead fisherman, Portland Trail Blazer fan, and Lutheran, who every few years extends her medical hand to refugees in Cambodia, Somalia,

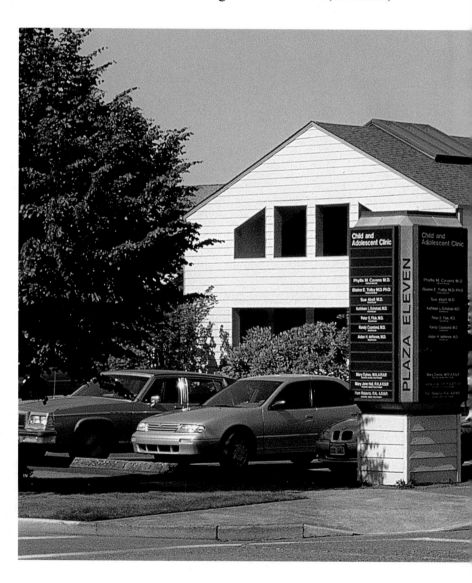

Ethiopia or Honduras. At this point in her life, she feels quite satisfied that she chose a career path that not only has led her to a position of community respect, but has allowed her to bond with generations of children as they grow up.

Becoming a pediatrician, however, is not an easy task. The first hurdle is to endure the stiff competition in college to gain acceptance to a medical school. This is followed by four years of medical education, and then three years in a pediatric residency program. Since the road is so long and hard, there has to be a deep motivation to choose it.

That motivation may stem from various desires — to heal; to be financially secure; or to be like doctors on TV.

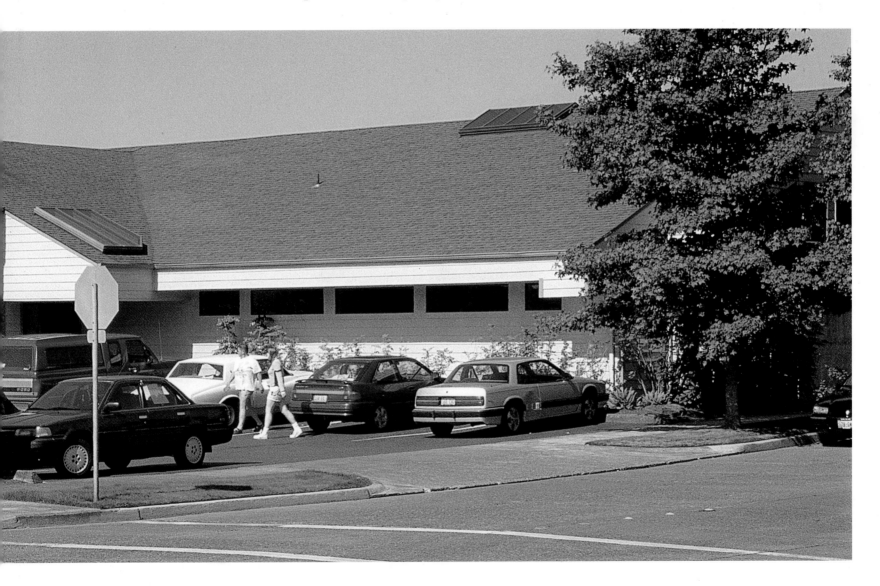

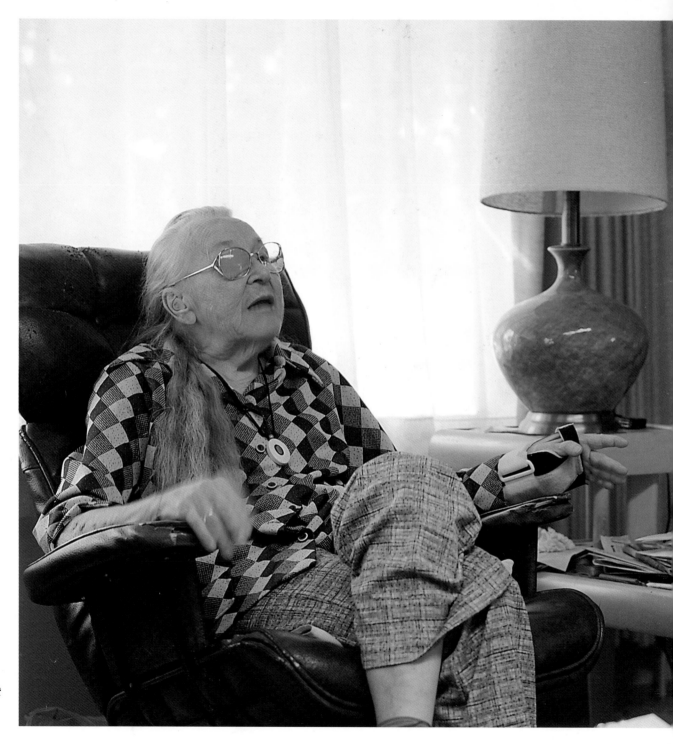

As Dr. Camilla Anderson, age 94, resumes her passionate attack on Freud, Dr. Phyllis Cavens confirms her own feelings that this dynamic psychiatrist was the inspiration that led her to enter medicine some 40 years earlier.

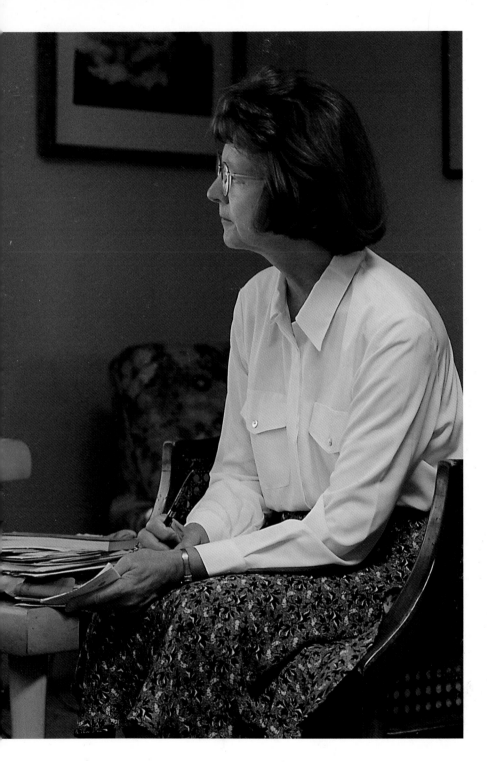

Sometimes a personal experience with medicine motivates aspiring pediatricians. They may have suffered as a child from a life-threatening disease that introduced them to the world of medicine. Or they may have been encouraged by a parent who was a doctor.

Others have no such private encounters, but are touched by someone outside their sphere who inspires them to dream of breaking though their self-imposed limitations to enter the field of medicine. This is the way it was for Phyllis Cavens. While a young woman, she met that someone who became her inspiration.

Meeting Her Inspiration

As a youngster growing up on a farm in Oregon, Phyllis never dreamed of going into medicine. She had, however, a "plotting" grandmother, Lena Larson.

Grandma Lena had taught grade school in Sydney, Montana, in 1910. One of her students was a bright little girl who grew up to become a psychiatrist and author, Dr. Camilla Anderson. Grandma arranged to invite Dr. Anderson to a private lunch at her home, along with Phyllis, who was just starting college.

Though Phyllis was not struck during this luncheon with a sudden revelation that caused her to shout out, "I want to be a doctor," she now realizes how pivotal that encounter was. It slowly opened her eyes to the possibility that she, too, could become a woman physician, and hopefully one as alive and vibrant as Dr. Anderson.

Four decades later in 1998, Phyllis and family members traveled to eastern Montana to once again meet her professional inspiration. Dr. Anderson was 94 years old at that time and was by her own reckoning, "falling apart." The fragile skin of her right arm was spotted with the vivid bruises of age, while the other arm, recently broken, was hidden by a Velcro splint. Her thinning gray hair could barely muster a semblance of a cascade over her shoulder.

And though she wore a patch over one eye, the other made sharp, commanding contact. Dr. Anderson gleefully held forth, at one point expounding on the philosophical nature of man and the need to support his feeling of "grandiosity," and the next, continuing her long fight against the teachings of Sigmund Freud. All those gathered around her were entranced.

As Phyllis listened, her long-held supposition was confirmed. This remarkable woman, who in her dotage could still captivate those around her, had been the one who awakened in her the nascent dream of becoming a physician.

The Road to The M.D. Degree

Phyllis's parents, Cliff and Viola Nyubakke, were Willamette Valley farmers who grew hops for making beer. Phyllis and her brother, John, worked in the fields, changing irrigation pipes and helping with the harvest. Though Viola was a college graduate who taught elementary school, Cliff, a Norwegian, had never finished grade school. But both valued education. When finances were low at one time, they sold the family piano to pay college tuition for Phyllis.

She graduated from Pacific Lutheran University in Tacoma, Washington, in 1961 and was accepted into the University of Oregon Medical School, one of only four women in a class of eighty. The women, enduring the male-dominated atmosphere, smiled weakly as the guys guffawed during class presentations by the anatomy professor whenever he used slides of Playboy centerfolds.

Phyllis and I were both in the same class. Our romance began in biochemistry lab, where we were seated across from each other. This led to a partnership on lab tests, and, as I've been telling people for years, "A certain intimacy grows when you are looking at each other's urine under the microscope."

That initial biochemical attraction led to marriage as soon as summer arrived. Two years later, we graduated from medical school in Portland, Oregon, and journeyed to Milwaukee, Wisconsin, for our rotating internship at Milwaukee County General Hospital.

It was hard. Not only were there long days in the hospital, but every third night we stayed overnight to care for patients, getting very little rest. A dormitory building was set aside for interns and residents, where they would try to snatch a few hours sleep between phone calls and emergency admissions. This dorm was just across the street from the hospital and connected by a short tunnel.

But Phyllis was not allowed to stay there — she was a woman. And even though we were married, she could not be assigned to my room. Instead, she had to go back and forth to the nurses' dorm, several blocks away, often trudging through the Midwest snow and cold. A tunnel from the nurses'

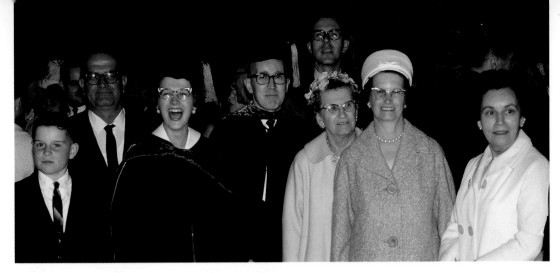

On the night of graduation from medical school an exuberant Phyllis Cavens, third from left, is flanked by her father, Cliff; her husband, myself; her grandmother, Lena; and her mother, Viola. **Family photo**

dorm to the hospital that once existed had been boarded up, because student nurses had been caught using it to go out on midnight romances.

After finishing our rotations on the pediatric ward, both Phyllis and I began to think that we should become pediatricians instead of family practitioners as we had originally planned. General medicine was too broad a field; we needed to specialize in one branch of medicine in order to be better prepared to handle the complicated cases and emergencies that were bound to occur. In addition, new technology had opened up the field of pediatrics with exciting medical advances, especially in the care of premature babies. But more importantly, we both liked children.

Starting a Small-Town Practice

We returned to Portland for our pediatric residency training, practiced in the city area for a few years and then moved to Longview because a position was available for me in a pediatric clinic. Since Phyllis had an additional year's train-

ing in treating handicapped children, she worked for a new program called Head Start and also for the Progress Center, a locally created service for developmentally delayed children. Eventually she was hired by the pediatric clinic where I practiced.

I was made a partner after one year, but clinic policy dictated that they would never take Phyllis in as a partner, unless one crucial requirement was met — that I died. This seemed to me to be asking for a bit much, so while I remained at that clinic, in 1978 Phyllis and another woman pediatrician, Dr. Sharon Hempler, started their own practice, the Child and Adolescent Clinic. There were lean times as the practice grew. Phyllis earned only $1,100 the first year.

Since that time, the clinic has expanded to a total of seven pediatricians and three pediatric nurse practitioners. It is a very busy place with a patient population of 15,000 children, generating more than 200 visits per day during the winter months.

It is a fast-paced life. In the following pages, I hope to give you a glimpse of the hectic day of a pediatrician with the stresses and joys that accompany it, using my wife, Dr. Phyllis Cavens, as the primary example.

2 ... in the hospital

A Crisis in the Delivery Room

I was awakened by the low, deep voice of my wife talking on the phone in the dark of our bedroom. She asked a rhetorical question, "So it's slow progress in labor?" — a pause — " I'll be right in." I opened my eyes to see the face of the alarm clock, which glowed "1:00" a.m. precisely. She slid from our bed and quietly closed the door behind her.

Dr. Phyllis Cavens was on her way to St. John Medical Center to yet another birth crisis. A mother was having a difficult labor, and the obstetrician needed to do a Caesarean section to get the baby out immediately. An order had been snapped: "Get the pediatrician."

I pictured my wife racing to the hospital in her Toyota Land Cruiser and knew that she was worried about the baby. Obviously there was a problem with the mother's labor, but Phyllis had been given no information over the phone about how the baby was doing. Was it just idly waiting to be born, or was it slowly suffocating in the mother's womb? As usual, she wouldn't know the details until she got there.

Even though she had already worked a full day at the clinic, and then seen an additional sixteen patients that evening because of influenza and respiratory syncytial virus epidemics, somehow she was ready to respond. The impending disaster had jolted her awake. Fortunately, this crisis resolved quickly when the baby emerged, crying lustily.

I opened my eyes once more when Phyllis slid back into bed. The clock read 2:27 a.m. She would get a few more hours' sleep before getting up at 6:30 for another C-section.

A Welcomed Son

The mother who was scheduled to have that next C-section was Nita Jones. I talked to her and her husband before the surgery to obtain their permission to photograph the delivery of their baby. They were a happy couple, excited about adding a new boy to their family. Father smiled enthusiasti-

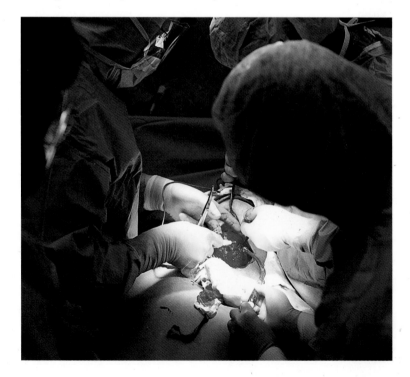

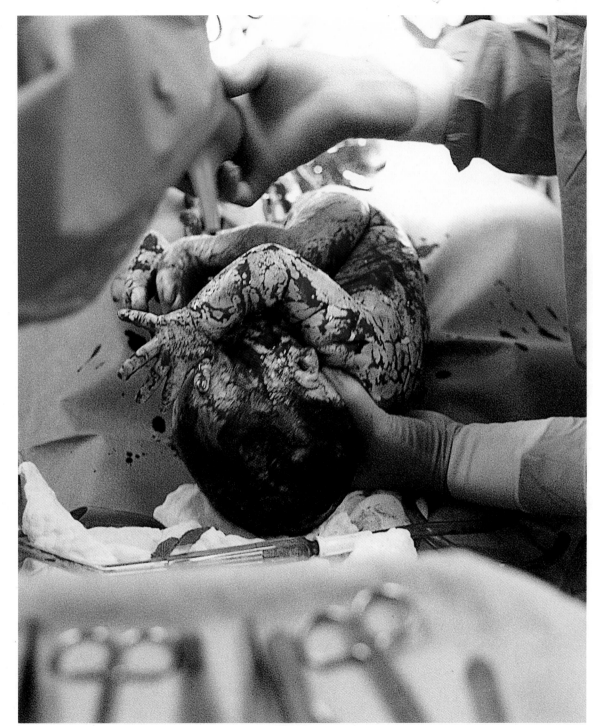

Far left: The obstetrician, Dr. Aris Gredzens, begins the Caesarean section on Nita Jones with an incision into her abdomen, using an electrocautery to control bleeding. Phyllis stands ready to suction the baby's mouth when it appears.

Right. The surgeon has handed the delivered baby to Phyllis, who once again clears its nose and throat of secretions with a suction bulb.

cally as he proudly explained that they would name him Miguel, but call him Migelito, for "little Miguel."

The father was allowed to be with his wife during the surgery. Dressed in green surgical scrubs, he was directed to sit behind a drape that obscured his view, but did allow him to comfort his wife. Having had an epidural block to anesthetize her from the waist down, she was awake as the surgery began.

Being an observer for the first time, rather than a participant, I was struck by how abruptly the chatter in the room stopped when the surgeon started to cut; there was only silence as all turned their attention to getting that baby out quickly.

When the obstetrician, Dr. Aris Gredzens, slid his fingers through the incision into the uterus to grasp the baby, the assistant surgeon put his hand on the mother's abdomen and pushed down. Suddenly, the baby's head popped into the bright light of the surgical field.

The baby lay there a few seconds, seemingly disembodied, while Phyllis quickly suctioned his mouth. Dr. Gredzens carefully pulled the rest of the tiny form out; the baby looked blue and bloody. There was a pause — a tense pause — as everyone waited for that first big cry of life. Finally it came and, as usual, it was surprisingly loud.

With a firm grip, Phyllis carried the wet, slippery newborn to an open-air stand that was warmed with radiant heat. While Phyllis and the nurse tended to the now-pink baby on the warmer, a delighted father leaned over to kiss his wife.

The Fragility of Birth

There is nothing more satisfying to the soul of a family than the birth of a baby. Each parent and grandparent, uncle and aunt, experience an exuberant emotion, based on a primal feeling — whether they realize it or not — that they are participating in their own immortality. Family members are excited as they see the new wonder for the first time, especially grandmothers, who are like flustered hens, bobbing up and down at the viewing widow.

It's exciting, too, for Phyllis, but from the far different perspective of an experienced pediatrician who knows that baby-making and birth are a fragile process. She can visualize all the changes inside a baby's heart and lungs as it suddenly surfaces from an all-water environment to air — changes that must go on within minutes as the lungs pop open for the first time, and the flow of blood seeks new pathways through the lungs and heart vessels.

Usually, birth goes miraculously well. But there are times when suddenly the whole process crashes; the obstetrician hands over a limp and blue baby, relieved to pass on the responsibility to the pediatrician.

The infant may not be breathing. The nurse quickly listens with a stethoscope and calls out the heart rate. As it falls, the pediatrician's heart rate inversely rises, bringing forth

Far right: A suction tube is passed through the throat of the baby into his stomach to clear amniotic fluid that would have been squeezed out if the baby had come normally through the birth canal. Nurse Sandi Archer carefully monitors the heart rate as the tube is passed.

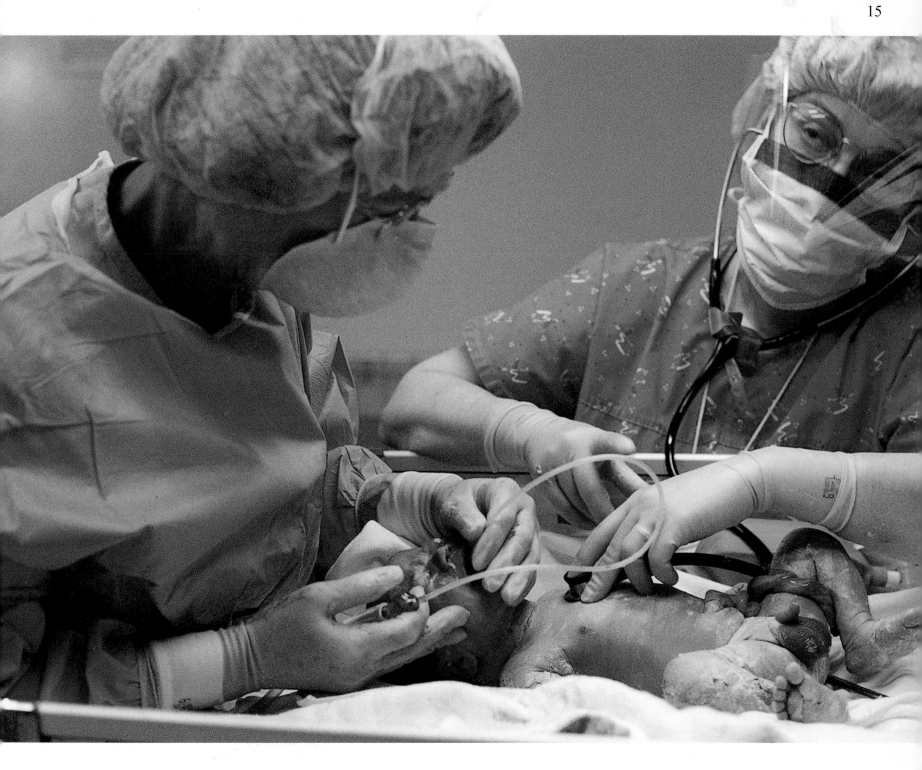

a well-rehearsed litany of action ... suction ... mask oxygen ... intubate ... chest massage ... adrenalin ... repeat.

A Perfect Baby

Fortunately, Migelito's birth went very well; there had been no need to resuscitate. As the surgeons were sewing Nita Jones back up after her C-section, Phyllis carried the baby to the nursery. His excited father strode quickly along with her, beaming with happiness.

As soon as the nurse measured Migelito's weight, length and head circumference, Phyllis completed a more detailed examination from head to toe. She assured the father that his baby was not just normal or OK, but perfect. Once again, he smiled broadly.

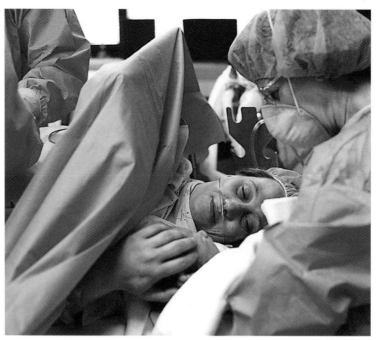

Nita Jones's new baby is positioned so that she can touch him and look into his eyes.

The Race to Resuscitate

The following is an abbreviated version of what typically happens when a fresh-born baby is in trouble:

NURSE ALERTS	PEDIATRICIAN'S THOUGHTS
"Baby not breathing."	*Look for color ... Is the chest rising ? ... Suction the throat.*
"Heart rate falling."	*Start bagging with oxygen ... Get a good seal with the mask.*
"Heart rate 80."	*Keep on bagging ... Still looks blue ... It's not breathing ... C'mon ... C'mon.*
"Heart rate 60."	*Got to tube the baby ... What size tube?*
"Heart rate 60."	*Begin chest massage ... Keep bagging ... Draw up adrenaline ... What dose? ... Must weigh 3 k.*
"Heart rate coming up."	*Can stop massage ... Still looks blue ... Keep on bagging.*
"Baby breathing."	*Wow, its pinking up. Let's get it to the nursery stat.* **"Everybody move."**
"Is it a boy or a girl?"	*Rats, I don't know; I haven't looked yet!*

Rounds on "Normal" Babies

Six other newborns awaited Phyllis that morning on her so-called "normal newborn" hospital rounds, but almost all of these "normal" babies had some sort of problem. Some were of a minor nature, but others were more serious. All of them would require careful examination and the analytical thinking of a pediatrician. Phyllis picked up a box containing some examination instruments, gathered the patient charts, and marched down the hall to begin.

Baby 1: Abnormal kidneys

Leaning over the crib of a baby boy, the doctor concentrated more than usual on examining his abdomen. The baby's skin was soft and warm as Phyllis slowly pressed her fingers down into his soft belly. She was hunting for something that she hoped would not be there — enlarged kidneys.

While he was still a fetus in the womb, an ultrasound imaging done on his mother had hinted that his kidneys were abnormally dilated. But the mysterious gray and white, blurry images of an ultrasound often are very hard to interpret. They could mean nothing, or they could be prebirth messengers warning that a congenital blocking of the urinary tract was forcing urine backwards into his bulging kidneys, slowly destroying them.

Phyllis couldn't feel big kidneys. That was a good sign, but it didn't completely rule out the possibility of a urinary-tract obstruction. She wrote an order for an ultrasound to be done on the baby, which would zoom in on his little abdomen. That test would answer the question as to whether the mother's ultrasound finding was an innocent fluke, or if life-threatening disease did exist. Both mother and doctor would have to be patient, however, since the results wouldn't be known until the next day.

Baby 2: Too small?

Even though the next baby in the room had been born after the usual 40 weeks of gestation, she weighed only five pounds, seven ounces. She was classified, therefore, as SGA, or small for gestational age. This is always a concern, leading the pediatrician to ponder why the baby is smaller than expected.

There can be many diverse reasons. The day before, Phyllis had studied the mother's health record to be sure that there was no history of prenatal infection or heavy use of drugs, alcohol or cigarettes as possible causes. There was none. Today, she was more concerned that the baby might have developed low blood sugar, since small infants often have inadequate reserves of carbohydrates stored in their liver.

She eyed the baby carefully, noting that the infant was alert and active. At the same time, there was no jitteriness — no little arms waving tremulously, as if begging for candy. That was a good sign. Phyllis leafed through the baby's chart, however, to find the glucose blood-test results. They would be more definitive. All of them were normal. Great! The baby, though small, was healthy. Phyllis felt safe in moving on to the next newborn.

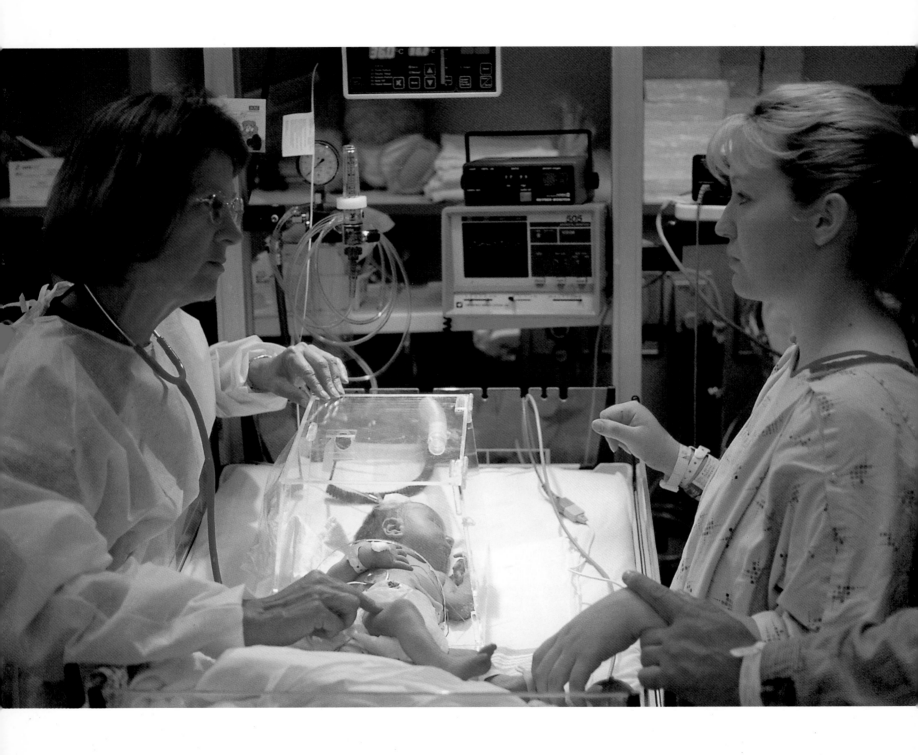

Baby 3: Was there heart disease?

Both mother and father of the next newborn were waiting for Phyllis. She knew them well, having helped them through the stress of coping with the congenital heart disease of their first child. Phyllis was fully aware that they were worried that this new baby might have heart problems also.

She placed her stethoscope on the baby's chest, just to the left of the sternum, and listened for a long time. She kept her head down, assuming that if she looked up, she would catch them intently watching her facial expression for clues as to whether the news was good or bad.

The tension grew as she repositioned the stethoscope further up the chest, listened some more, and then quickly moved it to the other side. She remained motionless, stethoscope tubing running from her ears to the little form in the bassinet.

Finally, she looked up and, knowing they needed to hear assurance, said with a firm voice, "If there is one thing I can tell you, your baby has a perfect heart. Babies that don't have a perfect heart have a murmur." There were smiles of relief.

Far left: Dr. Cavens discusses the progress of baby Gary Tussig with his mother, Kellie. Gary had difficulty breathing soon after birth which prevented him from eating. Intravenous fluids are being given to him through a small vein in his scalp and he is being kept warm by radiant heat from an overhead lamp. Extra oxygen flows into the plastic hood surrounding his head. A monitor attached to his left big toe measures the amount of oxygen getting into his blood stream and records his heart rate.

Baby 4: A real heart murmur

The baby in the next room, however, did have a murmur. An experienced nurse, Donna Boyle, had heard it first and reported it that morning. Phyllis once again positioned her stethoscope. There was indeed an abnormal "whooshing" noise, loud enough to pass through the ribs, cartilage and skin of the chest wall.

Phyllis analyzed the sound, listening to this possible whisper of insight concerning the blood-flow turmoil existing in the invisible, tiny recesses of the infant's heart. Either there was an innocent swirling of the blood through the heart chambers, signifying nothing, or blood was squirting through some abnormal hole. If that were true, the heart might already be straining to compensate and could eventually fail. There was no telling by just listening if or when that might occur.

An echocardiogram was needed. Phyllis planned to call an old friend of hers, a pediatric cardiologist in Portland, to bring his portable machine to Longview to do the test that day. But a problem loomed.

This baby's insurance program didn't have that cardiologist on its panel. The echocardiogram would have to be done by another doctor who didn't travel and who usually turned down requests for immediate appointments in Portland.

Dr. Cavens was irritated, for she was going to have to push hard to get the second-choice pediatric cardiologist to see the child, even within the next week. Managed care was once again needlessly endangering a patient and prolonging the anxiety of parents in order to save dollars.

Baby 5: A C-section baby

The next patient was a baby delivered by C-section the day before. There were no apparent problems in feeding or voiding, so Phyllis began a routine evaluation of the social situation. With gentle questioning, she determined that the baby was going home to a safe environment with good family support.

She proceeded to teach the current pediatric litany — place your baby on her back for sleeping; use a car safety seat; don't smoke around your baby; check your smoke detector; and bring your baby into the office in two days. These many topics had to be covered quickly, since managed care pushed mothers and babies out of the hospital more rapidly than before.

Baby 6: The confrontation

The family in the next room presented a real challenge. Mother and Grandma were there to take on the doctor.

They wanted the baby to go home on a monitor that would watch his breathing and set off an alarm if it stopped. They were afraid of SIDS, or Sudden Infant Death Syndrome, because they thought their baby had turned blue in the night.

Dr. Phyllis explained that years ago it was believed that apnea spells, in which babies stopped breathing for short periods, led to SIDS, but current research had disproved that theory. As of today, no one knows what causes SIDS, but doctors are sure that having a monitor on the child doesn't prevent the tragedy. The two women didn't buy that.

The mother raised the argument to a higher pitch; then as Dr. Cavens attempted to educate her, the young woman ran out of steam and drifted to the other side of the room. Grandma took over. She rose from her chair, crossed her arms and stared directly into Phyllis's face as she claimed loudly that many, many of their family members had apnea that required monitors.

The harangue went on for many minutes with Dr. Cavens trying to keep her voice low and authoritative. She knew that they were acting out of anxiety and lack of trust, because they had just met her and had no past history by which to judge her intention to help them.

As a compromise, she offered to keep the baby for an additional night, do some tests, and watch him on a monitor during that time. Grandma accepted this, and the confrontation came to a sputtering close.

Phyllis then glanced at the new mother in the next bed, a patient of a doctor from a different clinic. Phyllis wondered what that mother's impression was of the whole tirade.

Worries on the Pediatric Ward

After finishing rounds in the nursery, Phyllis went up one flight of stairs to the pediatric ward to check on three children that she had hospitalized 72 hours earlier. All of them were very worrisome cases.

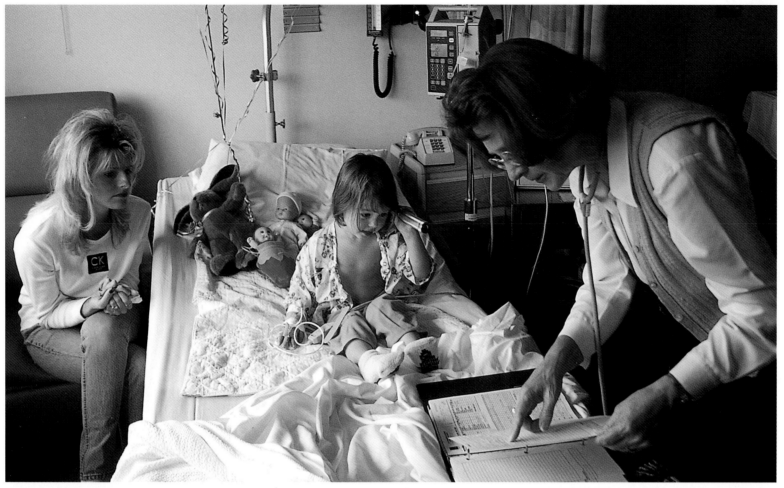

For a week, 4-year-old Madelynn Martin suffered from the usual symptoms of influenza. But on the night she was admitted to the hospital with a high fever, she was grunting as she fought to breathe. On this morning, Dr. Cavens sees that Madelynn is markedly improved. While she studies the nurses' notes and laboratory reports to confirm her clinical observations, the little girl's mother, Michaele Martin, anxiously waits for word that her daughter can go home soon. (Phyllis was able to discharge her little patient later that evening.)

... a 2-month-old with pneumonia

An infant boy had been directly admitted from the clinic with pneumonia. This pneumonia was more serious than the usual little patch of infection showing up as a wisp of white on the chest Xray. This was lobar pneumonia. A solid section of white on the film revealed an entire lobe of lung filled with pus. The child's precarious existence was even more threatened, because he had been born prematurely and was barely two months old.

An IV had been started in a tiny vein, allowing big doses of an antibiotic that Phyllis had chosen that first day. But running in the back of her mind since then had been the constant question, "Will the antibiotic do its job and kill the bacteria?"

As she looked at the baby this morning, she felt the anxiety of the last few days disappear. The baby looked better; there was no fever or labored breathing. Since the pulse oximeter showed normal oxygen levels, she mustered up the courage to take the next step and ordered the nurse to try weaning the baby off his oxygen. If that went well during the next few hours, he might even go home tonight, she thought. Ah, sweet success....

... a problem in diagnosis

Phyllis next stood at the fold-down desk in the hallway, reviewing the chart of a 4-month-old girl who came in with high fever, vomiting and diarrhea. Today's lab test was positive for rotavirus, which might explain the illness. However, there was a second possibility.

This baby had a past history of urine backing up from her bladder into her kidneys, causing repeated infections. Was this reflux the cause of the fever this time? Since the baby had been given an antibiotic before admission to the hospital, it wasn't possible to rely on the usual urine culture test to see if infection was present.

There was, therefore, no exact way to know whether the rotavirus infection or a kidney problem was the cause of the fever. When doctors are faced with this dilemma, they often decide, as Phyllis did, to treat both possibilities.

But that wasn't what bothered Phyllis this morning. The nurse informed her that the family doctor had dropped by and had been critical of collecting the urine specimen by inserting a rubber catheter into the bladder. He told the mother that a needle should have been stuck directly through the abdomen into the baby's bladder to suck out the urine to get a purer sample.

Dr. Cavens knew that the mother would now wonder about which doctor to trust and would worry about whether her baby was getting the best care.

Before Phyllis entered the room, she rehearsed in her mind what she was going to say to the mother. She would explain that pediatricians believe that bladder needle sticks are old-fashioned.

As the mother listened to Phyllis and thought about what her baby might have gone through, she readily accepted the pediatrician's approach.

... a baby exuding pus; the spinal tap

The patient in the next room, a 5-week-old girl, had been even more worrisome — and still was. The infant's trouble had started when a thick, oily layer of scales formed a cradle cap of the scalp, which had become infected. The infection had spread, causing pus to ooze from her ears, vagina, and folds of skin. Her temperature was 101. She was admitted to the hospital with the very real possibility that bacteria may well have invaded her blood or spinal fluid.

This automatically called for an immediate spinal tap. Such a procedure demands the slow insertion of a needle between the tiny bony projections of the back that protect the small fluid-filled tube, the spinal canal. It's a narrow-enough target in an adult, but much, much smaller in a baby. The doctor can easily miss and hit a blood vessel, drawing blood rather than the sought-for spinal fluid.

The nurse, Debbie Nida, placed the baby on her side on a bedside table that had been adjusted to Phyllis's eye level. The doctor then encouraged Debbie to get a good grip on the baby's shoulders and hips to fold her small form into a tight little ball.

Phyllis swabbed the bowed back with Betadyne and injected some anesthetic. She now imagined her target, aiming the needle towards the belly button. As it slid through the narrow bony opening, the baby struggled and cried, but Debbie kept the infant girl in line.

The pediatrician, moving her hand very slowly, could sense with her fingers the progress of the needle as it went through the tissues. Finally she felt, more than heard, a "pop" as the point entered the spinal tube. The clear fluid that dripped from the needle hub was sent stat to the lab, which confirmed that there was no meningitis. That was a relief.

But what was going on? Did the baby have a generalized infection of her bloodstream with bacteria being seeded into every crevice of her body, or was this merely an infected cradle cap? Phyllis took no chances. After the spinal tap, she ordered IV antibiotics that would treat the most virulent staph infection.

Now, days later, as Phyllis bent over to examine the baby, she saw that her patient was acting much better and eating well. The drainage of pus had stopped, and there was no fever.

But certain fears still gnawed at Phyllis as they had earlier in the week. Had the baby been treated with enough IV Vancomycin to kill any staph-resistant bacteria in the baby's blood? Could she trust today's lab report that the staph was indeed sensitive to the antibiotic? Why did the baby still have this bright red rash? And finally, she struggled with the most important question: Was it safe to send the baby home today on oral antibiotics as planned?

The baby's mother was at the crib, waiting for a decision. Dr. Cavens had to act, one way or the other, as doctors do many times a day. She finally said with professional confidence, "Your baby can go home, but you must keep her on the antibiotic, and I want to see her tomorrow." The mother smiled with happiness.

Phyllis left the hospital at eleven a.m. The past 28 hours had been tiring due to long hours, lack of sleep, and a heavy load of complex patients. This doesn't happen every day, but it does occur fairly frequently in the life of a pediatrician.

That's what makes it exciting and meaningful.

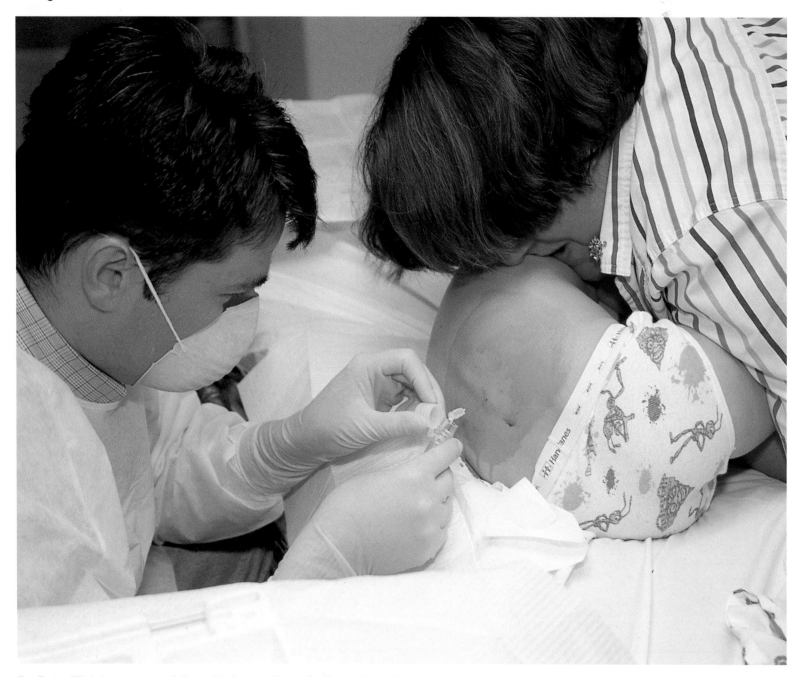

Dr. Peter Filuk has successfully guided a small needle through the bony projections of Brian Schatzel's back to enter the tiny spinal canal. Clear fluid is seen dripping from the spinal needle into a collection tube. This will be sent immediately to the lab to exclude meningitis as a cause of the child's fever and headache.

Treating the Physician's Son

There was more tension than usual one evening for Dr. Peter Filuk, a partner in the Child and Adolescent Clinic, when he faced the responsibility of treating 4-year-old Brian. This little boy, the son of clinic partner Dr. Kathleen Schatzel, had a 104-degree fever and a severe headache. The combination of these symptoms indicated the need to do a spinal tap.

Pediatricians dread these situations when they must care for the child of another physician, knowing that their medical colleague has similar knowledge about what should be done. But at the same time, they also realize that their partner is like any other parent when their child is very sick; they desperately want to hear the voice of medical authority.

Dr. Filuk responded well, moving ahead to do the tap, apparently calm. But he had additional stress to deal with. There would be two pediatricians watching his every move. I would be in the room taking repeated pictures with my camera, and the child's mother, Dr. Schatzel, would be holding her son during the procedure.

It went well, with clear spinal fluid dripping into the collection tube with the first pass of the needle. And Brian held very still, soothed by his mother's embrace and soft words. There was relief among the three of us pediatricians and the usual congratulatory, "Good shot, Doctor."

The laboratory found no meningitis in the spinal fluid.

As David Schatzel helps in comforting his son after the spinal tap, Brian's mother reassures him that he did very well.

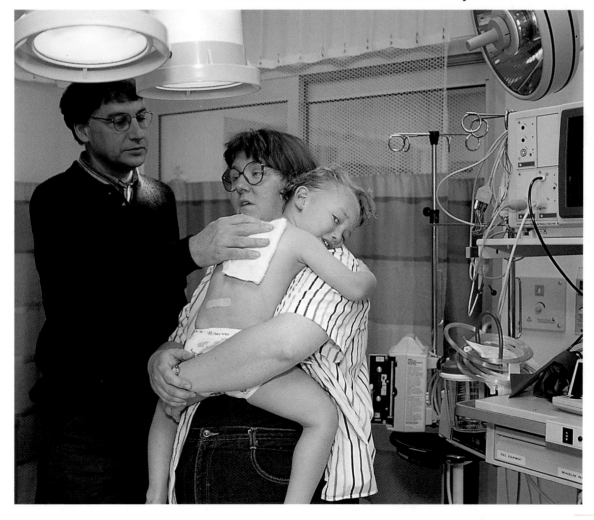

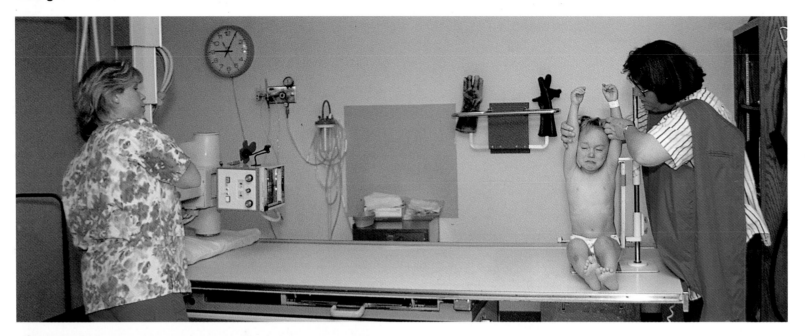

Above: While a side view of his chest is being taken by the radiology technician, Brian's mother holds his arms up so those bones don't show up in the Xray of his lungs.

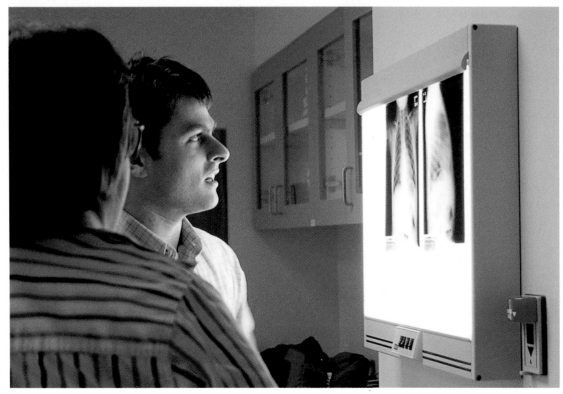

Left: Dr. Peter Filuk studies Brian's Xray for possible pneumonia as a cause of his high fever and headache. None is found.

Patient Epilogue

Baby 1 — abnormal kidneys? (page 17). The baby whose mother's ultrasound showed him to have enlarged kidneys underwent his own ultrasound the next day. It was normal.

Baby 4 — a heart murmur (page 19). The baby with the murmur saw a pediatric cardiologist seven days later and had no heart disease.

Baby 6 — the confrontation (page 20). The mother and grandmother, who had been worried about apnea, felt satisfied the next day that overnight monitoring had been normal. They listened attentively as Phyllis went through the routine instructions of taking care of a baby at home. She had earned their trust.

The observing mother (page 20). The mother in the next bed, who had witnessed their tirade, later called the office to switch care of her baby to Phyllis.

... a baby exuding pus (page 22). The 5-week-old with fever, rash, and pus who had the spinal tap was seen the next day in clinic and was well.

The physician's son (page 25). Brian continued to worry his parents and clinic doctors for a full seven days with a 103- to 105-degree fever. He then recovered fully from his viral illness.

Two Advances in Pediatrics

... the butterfly needle

In order to get blood from children for tests or to treat them with lifesaving fluids and drugs, a pediatrician must be able to get a needle into the vein or artery of a child. Since the blood vessels of toddlers and babies are so small, this was almost impossible years ago. The large-bore needles that were originally created for adults were much too big.

Smaller versions were eventually manufactured, but these delicate needles were very difficult to grasp between a forefinger and thumb, and accurately poke them into hidden, little veins. In addition, once inserted in the vessel, they wouldn't stay in place very long. A very simple solution to this problem was conceived in the 1960s.

Two little plastic wings were attached at the base of a tiny needle. These half-inch tabs were flexible and allowed the doctor to firmly grasp the needle as he guided the sharp point through the skin and into the vessel. And once inside the vein, tape could be applied to the wings to hold the needle still. Because of their winged appearance, they were nicknamed "butterfly" needles.

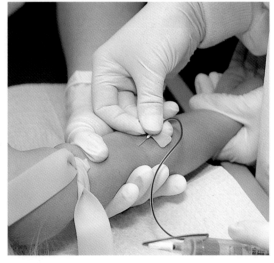

With a nurse holding a child's arm, a laboratory technician draws blood from a vein, holding onto one wing of the butterfly needle to steady it.

Butterfly needles revolutionized pediatrics. Now children could be treated for shock and given antibiotics quickly, plus premature babies could receive long-term nourishment through IV care. And pediatricians, armed with this new development, finally became recognized as skilled experts.

... Caesarean section

Another development in medicine that has helped children live better lives is the more widespread use of Caesarean section. The obstetrician is more inclined to use this surgical means of delivery if trouble is looming.

Phyllis recalls that at the start of her career, there were more battered babies born because there was a desire back then to deliver the "natural" way. But "nature" can be cruel,

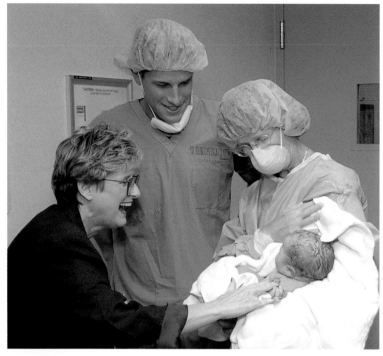

and babies can come out neurologically damaged. A timely C-section, however, often prevents such tragedies. Dr. Phillip Henderson wisely decided to deliver the baby of John and Jenna Anderson (pictured) by this route.

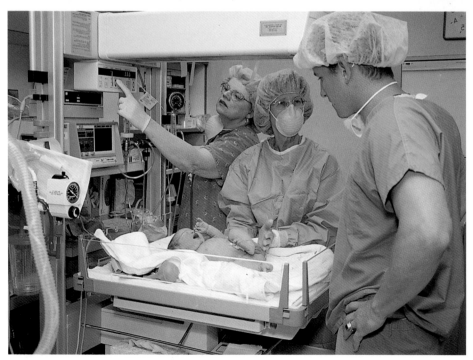

Above: Pat Anderson experiences by touch the exuberance of being a grandmother, while her son John Anderson beams with pride. He and Dr. Cavens have just emerged from the surgical suite where his baby was delivered by C-section.

Left: While nurse Sandi Nolden adjusts the radiant heater, Dr. Cavens reassures Mr. Anderson that he has a perfect baby girl.

Far right: Jenna Anderson blissfully relaxes as baby Marley gets a final discharge examination.

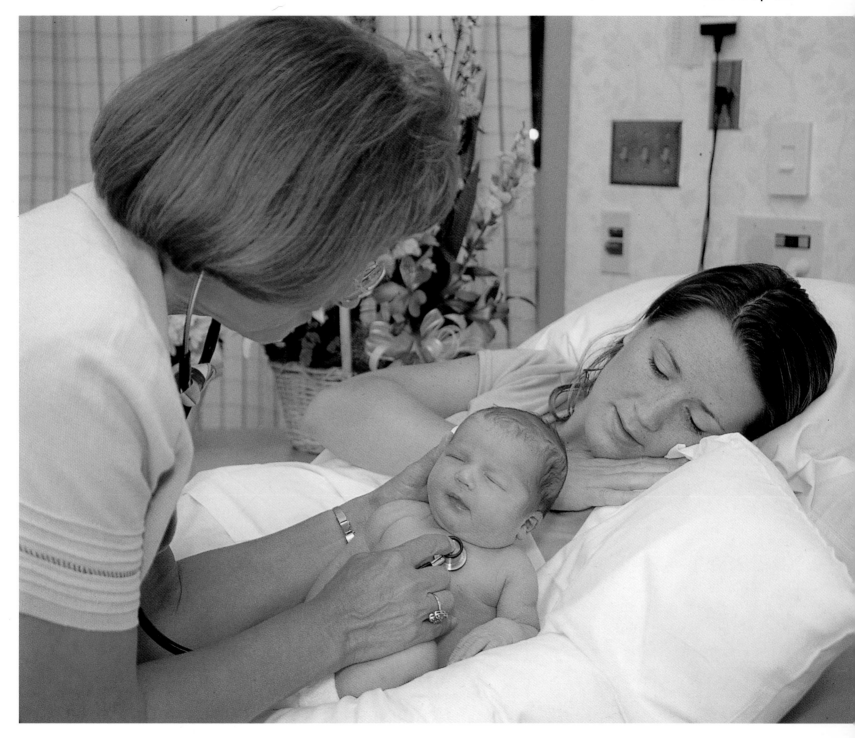

3 ... in the clinic

Opening That Door

Each day in the clinic, the pediatrician begins seeing patients by opening an exam room door and stepping inside his or her eight-by-ten-foot cubicle. At that point, neither the doctor, the patient, nor the parent can easily escape the ensuing encounter.

And the visits are always so different — the patient varies; the parent varies; the disease varies. A 2-year-old patient might greet the doctor with a howl of fright or a running embrace of happiness. The teenager may grin a friendly "Hi" or sit sullen, daring anyone to elicit words.

The parents may have a list of intelligent questions on their minds to be asked with thankful civility, or they may be sitting, tight-lipped, ready to launch a verbal attack due to some perceived slight. Pediatrics is never dull.

Tougher Cases

A variety of children will present themselves to the doctor each day, but there has been a marked change in the last 10 years in the types of patients seen. No longer are pediatricians just treating colds and diaper rashes or simply discussing the introduction of baby foods. Today, they take care of far more complex patients.

The simpler problems of children are now solved in other ways. Parents can get medical advice from books or the Internet. Many medicines that formerly required a prescription can be purchased "over the counter." A busy mother can now treat her child's cold, cough, fever, pain, head lice, diaper rash, eczema, impetigo, hives, ringworm, or diarrhea without a visit to the doctor.

If the child's illness is slightly more worrisome, the mother might obtain telephone help from an advice nurse at the office or make an appointment with a nurse practitioner. Thus, the relatively easy medical problems are more frequently treated by someone other than a physician. This leaves a greater number of more serious and complicated cases to be channeled to the pediatrician.

This was amply illustrated one particular day in the life of Dr. Phyllis Cavens. That day was **December 17.**

December 17

When Phyllis came home from work that Thursday evening, she lamented to me about the difficulties of the day. She was tired; it had been very busy. But it was also a fairly typical day for a pediatrician — one of barely controlled chaos. Since December 17 appeared to be so representative, I chose it to be a "Rosetta stone" for translating the daily life of a children's doctor.

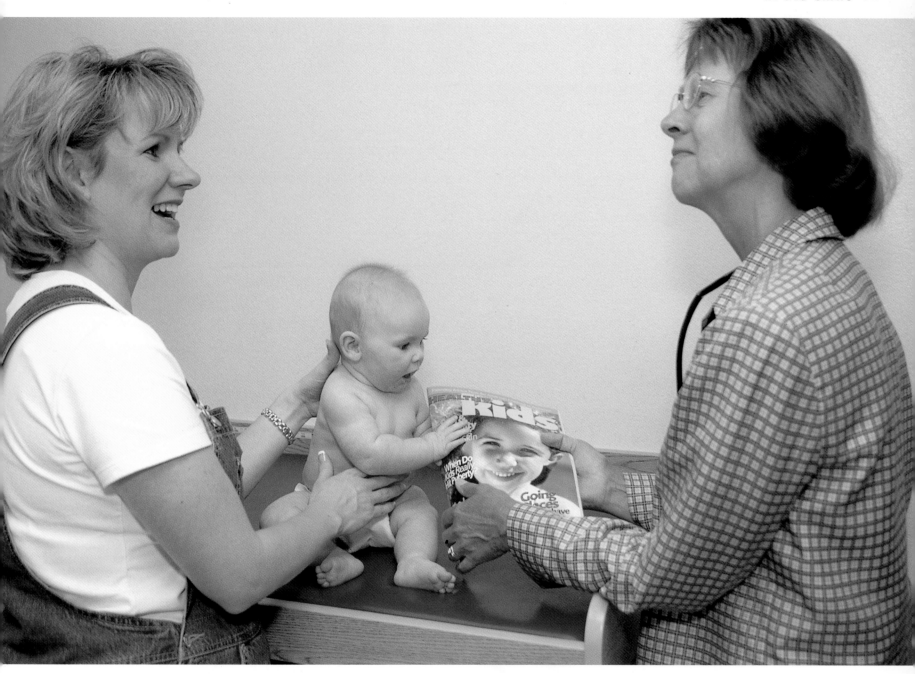

Six-month-old Brook Richter appears precociously interested in Healthy Kids, *a magazine published by the American Academy of Pediatrics, as her mother and Dr. Cavens discuss her development and diet. The magazine is given free to parents during well-child examinations.*

All the charts of that one day were gathered, and I took notes as Phyllis recalled her encounters with each child. As I wrote first of one patient and then the next one, that day began to unfold before my eyes. It became obvious that pediatric practice is not just colds, earaches and diaper rashes.

Instead, there were children with profound psychiatric problems, and youngsters trying to survive in dysfunctional families. There were patients with chronic diseases that required up-to-date knowledge of their pathology and of the newest medicines. There were children who needed not only leadership in obtaining special services for their problems, but also help in penetrating the barriers that insurance companies had thrown up.

That day, **December 17**, began with a morning parade of problems.

December 17 — morning

Since Phyllis was working mornings in the hospital nursery that week, she was scheduled to start seeing patients in the clinic at 10:00 a.m., rather than 9, but there had been an unforeseen problem in getting care for a premature baby. She was late, therefore, for the first appointment.

She glanced at the patient schedule taped above her desk. This simple-appearing list of complaints did not begin to convey the reality of the complex problems that faced her. But first, there were five phone calls to respond to.

Phyllis recognized most of the names on the list of phone messages and cringed, knowing that several of the patients had difficult diseases to manage, and that their parents were even more difficult. She wrote some return messages on each and rose to start seeing her waiting patients.

... in need of a psychiatrist

Upon entering the exam room of **Patient 1**, she noted that the young adolescent had been scheduled for a quick "med check" with the single purpose of refilling a Ritalin prescription. This seemed easy, so she had some expectation of catching up on her schedule. That hope was shattered, however, when she opened the 13-year-old's thick chart and recalled that his multiple behavior problems required him to take, not just one, but four brain-altering, psychiatric medicines, each of them three times a day.

Because the patient's insurance coverage had been changed to public assistance, he could no longer see the psychiatrist who had started this cornucopia of medicines. Prescribing this mix of potent drugs with conflicting side effects was a job that required a psychiatrist, but the other psychiatrists in town had also turned the boy down over the last few months.

Phyllis decided to press the staff at a psychiatric center to see him. Opening the exam room door to beckon the nurse, she instructed her to call the center and bluntly tell the staff that the boy was coming to their place today for help, appointment or no appointment. In addition, Phyllis ordered the receptionist to fax over his records, wanted or not.

Phyllis then turned to the boy's mother to firmly instruct her to go to the center now with the referral form in her hand. "Don't go home first. Don't go eat. Go now."

Phyllis felt some regret about marshaling all these forces and pushing, but this adolescent needed help. His complex mental disturbances and depression put him at risk for suicide.

... teaching asthma control

Leaving the details for her staff to finish, she quickly turned to the next exam room to greet **Patient 2**, a 4-year-old boy with asthma. This disease is one that frightens both the patient and those around them. As a child with asthma struggles to breathe, it is as if an iron fist were squeezing their chest.

But Phyllis had taught this child's parents how to use an asthma inhaler. When their son started coughing two days before, they took the inhaler and hooked it up to a "spacer," a device that gathers all the puffs of medicine released from the inhaler and gets it into the child's lungs.

It had worked. There was no wheezing now. Phyllis reassured his mother that she was doing a good job, and finished by writing a prescription for one of the new 24-hour antihistamines to dry up his nose.

... a case of scarlet fever

An experienced glance at the red rash of the next child, **Patient 3**, told Dr. Cavens that he probably had scarlet fever due to strep throat. But doctors like to be as sure as possible in making a diagnosis, so a rapid strep test was ordered. It indeed showed a strep infection that would respond well to amoxicillin.

But the ensuing conversation with the child's father, who was so likable, caused Phyllis some remorse. He asked her to write a prescription for him, too, since he felt a sore throat coming on.

She looked at him, wanting to do him this favor and save him time in his busy day. By all odds, he too had strep, and it would have been so easy for her to scribble out one more prescription. But, with her voice pitched slightly higher, she politely explained that he should see his own doctor who knew his medical history and was responsible for his health.

This was the proper medical pathway. Still, she wondered if she was being too rigid in sticking to the usual guidelines. It was hard to turn him down, but he made no objection. He really was a very nice father.

... a simple physical

The next two patients had been scheduled for routine well-child checkups, with no particular problems being mentioned. The complete examination of **Patient 4** required several preliminary steps that are often hard for a 4-year-old. But the little girl quickly demonstrated good vision by correctly pointing her finger in the same direction as the "table legs" of the Big E on the wall chart were aimed.

During the hearing test, she laughingly dropped poker chips into a bucket whenever she heard the smallest sound coming from the headphones that engulfed the sides of her head. She could hear very well. The clinic aide then urged her to stand on the tremulous scale to measure her weight and height.

Finishing the basic measurements of vision, hearing, height and weight, the aide turned to her and requested the most bewildering, embarrassing thing: "Please pee in this cup." With the help of her mother, she was able to comply.

As Phyllis came into the room and greeted her, she noted the child's charming, reciprocal social skills. Other signs of mental development were normal, as was the physical examination. The little girl would do well in kindergarten, but the pediatrician covered a half dozen topics with mother and daughter to increase the chances of her being a successful and healthy student: wear a seat belt ... use a bicycle helmet ... have a fire drill ... limit TV ... go to bed at a regular time ... eat breakfast ... get a library card ... read together.

... a child with Tourette Syndrome

The scheduled routine exam for **patient 5**, however, was far from "routine." In addition to all the procedures of the well-child check, this 7-year-old boy needed a review of his malady, Tourette Syndrome or TS. He was on medicine to keep his odd behaviors, called tics, under control.

Children with TS are often helpless to control sudden twitches of their face, or they may voice random guttural sounds. Some patients may shock those around them by punctuating the air with staccato-driven obscenities, completely unintended.

Phyllis asked if the prescribed medicine was having side effects and if it was preventing the boy from embarrassing himself or those around him. His mother smilingly responded that it was working well.

... an antibiotic reaction

Patient 6 was a 9-month-old girl who had been treated for pneumonia with an oral antibiotic. The baby now had a bad diaper rash. While the potent medicine had cleared the lung infection, it had also killed off normal skin bacteria, allowing yeast to invade her bottom. Dr. Cavens prescribed a cream for this.

But the visit was not over. Phyllis took time to review the baby's immunization record, finding that the little girl needed a hepatitis B shot. Every visit nowadays, whether well or sick, is a chance to catch up on a missing immunization.

... a resilient girl with adrenal problems

Phyllis next walked into the room of **Patient 7**, and greeted 9-year-old Brooke Galloway with a big smile of familiarity. Brooke, a pretty little girl, had a rare disease called adrenal insufficiency.

Her adrenal glands didn't make enough of a particular hormone that is designed to keep sodium or salt from being lost in the urine. If her sodium dropped too low, she could quickly go into shock.

Phyllis had diagnosed the problem years before when 2-week-old Brooke was admitted to the hospital because of poor sucking and no weight gain. A blood sample then showed a dangerously low sodium level that Phyllis countered with a push of IV fluids containing salt and a high dose of hydrocortisone.

Brooke took medicine daily now to replace what her adrenal glands didn't produce. But oral substitution is crude, lacking the quick response of normal-functioning adrenal glands to stress and infection.

In 1998, Brooke was rushed to Legacy Emanuel Hospital's intensive care unit in Portland, Oregon, because of vomiting and poor responsiveness. Her sodium was dangerously low, but once again, she recovered, proving that she was indeed a fighter.

This day's visit was about ab-dominal pain, coupled with a craving for table salt and pickles with their salty brine. Since sodium is a principal ingredient in salt, there was concern that her body was sending a message to her appetite center that her sodium might be dangerously low once again. Phyllis reviewed her chart, examined her and ordered the needed blood work. Fortunately, the sodium test came back completely normal. Mother was relieved; doctor was relieved.

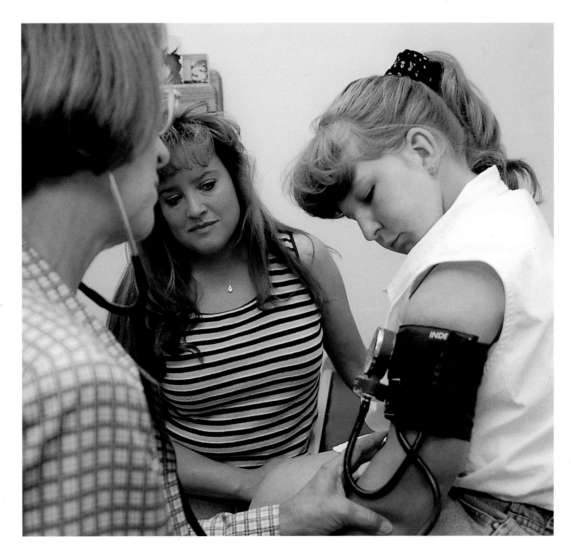

While her mother watches, Brooke Galloway, a plucky girl with adrenal problems, carefully monitors the taking of her blood pressure.

... a missing mother

Patient 8 was a child who had just been diagnosed with Attention Deficit Syndrome with Hyperactivity, known as ADHD. The purpose of the visit was to discuss the reasons for making the diagnosis and the proposed treatment with Ritalin. The side effects of that drug needed to be outlined as well as the follow-up school reports and doctor visits. In addition, the usual appointment with a psychologist needed to be arranged.

Unfortunately Phyllis had to give all this information to the child's grandmother, since his mother was in jail.

... a fragile asthmatic

The pediatrician's mental processing automatically jumped a few gigabytes when she realized that **Patient 9** was Ryan Stariha, a 4-year-old boy who five months earlier had been near death from asthma.

He had been rushed by ambulance to Doernbecher Children's Hospital with impending respiratory failure. There, a medicine was given by IV to open his severely constricted airways, but a side effect sent his heart beating so fast it could not pump his blood effectively. Another counteracting drug was quickly administered, saving his life.

Though he had come in today with the simple complaint of "cough," Phyllis was fully aware that his health stakes were much higher. She carefully examined Ryan, finding with relief that his lungs were clear. She then reviewed the four

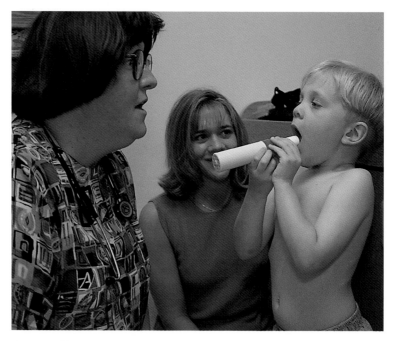

During a follow-up visit three weeks later, Dr. Kathleen Schatzel, his usual pediatrician, coaches Ryan Stariha to blow as hard as he can into a peak flowmeter to measure how his lungs are working.

asthma medicines he was taking and was pleased that he wouldn't be using any steroids this time. He was stable. After prescribing an antibiotic for a sinus infection, she smiled goodbye.

... a squeeze-in

Phyllis was late for the start of the clinic's weekly noon business meeting, but the practice of medicine is never orderly. The nurse approached her, almost apologetically, knowing that she was bringing news of an irritating situation. A mother had just arrived unannounced from the hospital emergency room demanding that her girl be seen now.

The wait had been too long at the ER, so she had left abruptly. The mother couldn't be told to come back to the clinic later, since her child did have a chronic condition that sometimes became suddenly serious, and there was no way to know if this was one of those times.

Phyllis sighed and instructed the nurse to get **patient 10** into a room immediately. She did an examination detailed enough to assure herself and the mother that the child was OK this time around. The harried doctor then rushed into the doctors' meeting room 45 minutes late for the noon meeting. But her partners also were slow in seeing their last patients; the meeting was yet to start.

December 17 — afternoon

... the sutures give way

Chin lacerations in a toddler are tough to sew up. **Patient 11** had been to the ER earlier where the doctor there had chased his evasive chin with needle and thread.

Phyllis saw him two days later when the active life of this 3-year-old had forced the wound to pop through the stitches, leaving it gaping. She explained to his mother that it would be a useless struggle to try to sew it again, because the edges of old lacerations don't stick together. The cut would still slowly heal, but with a slightly wider scar. All the doctor could do at this time was tape the cut to keep it clean.

... a trusting baby

As Phyllis entered the next exam room, she greeted **patient 12,** a 6-month-old boy, with the exaggerated speech used in addressing all infants, "Hello, t-h-e-e-e-r-e, how are y-o-o-o-u?"

The boy smiled back, an appropriate social response for his age. In addition, Phyllis noted he was sitting up by himself, another milestone in development. As she approached the happy baby, he showed no fear of her. In his young innocence, he didn't know that she was the one who would order the shots after she finished his well-baby exam.

Though an extra five minutes is scheduled for well-baby appointments, Phyllis still felt rushed as she covered the assigned topics of the 6-month exam. She talked about the prevention of poisoning and then demonstrated how to perform a baby Heimlich maneuver, hoping her efforts would spare this sparkling child from a possible disaster in the future.

... from baby fat to adolescent bulk

She was startled when she faced **patient 13**, a child who had been under her care since he was a baby. But now, towering before her was a muscular 16-year-old who weighed 180 pounds. She spoke to him, not with her baby voice, but with a "Hey dude, how's it going?" attitude.

He needed a routine sports physical to play soccer. But as often happens, his visit was not "routine." Not only was it necessary to review his allergy medicines, but his asthma status needed to be tested too. Phyllis had him blow as hard as he could into a peak flow meter. The results were good, so no changes in medicine were needed. But before he got out the door, she made sure that he got his needed diphtheria-tetanus and hepatitis shots.

... is there pneumonia?

The mother of **patient 14** was worried that her 15-month-old girl had been coughing for four days. After examining her baby's throat and ears, Phyllis listened intently with her stethoscope for any bubbles of fluid in the lungs. There was none. All that was needed was reassurance of no bronchitis or pneumonia, and a goodbye smile.

... repeated ear infections

Patient 15 was a 3-year-old boy. He and his mother had been in so many times with his ear infections that Phyllis greeted them as old friends. The child had been scheduled for surgery to have little plastic tubes put in his eardrums, the most commonly performed surgery in the United States nowadays, but that was several weeks away. So Phyllis prescribed enough antibiotic to prevent pain and fever until the ear-nose-and-throat doctor did his job.

... a smiling boy in spite of cerebral palsy

Patient 16 also was like an old friend with many shared experiences. Nathan Noss had started life in a battle to survive. He was born 11 weeks early, weighing only 2 pounds, 9 ounces. As he grew, he had to endure multiple surgeries and hospitalizations.

He was now age 16 and needed a wheelchair, but Nathan always had a happy smile whenever Dr. Cavens entered the exam room. Their light banter back and forth was based on years of knowing each other.

At this visit, he was being rechecked for a pneumonia, but he was more excited about getting to go to a professional wrestling match in Tacoma. It was his Christmas present. Phyllis asked him, "Nathan, do you know about the new governor of Minnesota?" "Oh, yeah," he replied, "that's Jesse Ventura, a wrestler. He's great."

... a urinary tract infection

Patient 17 was a teen-age girl who had pain with urination. Her symptoms and age dictated testing for sexually transmitted disease, but none was found. Her urine, however, showed pus cells swimming around, evidence of a common urinary tract infection. Phyllis prescribed a sulfa drug.

... a boy with depression

When Phyllis entered the next room, she was met by a 15-year-old boy, **patient 18**, who had deep emotional prob-

Opposite: Dr. Cavens gives Nathan Noss the thumbs-up sign for his continuing enthusiasm for life.

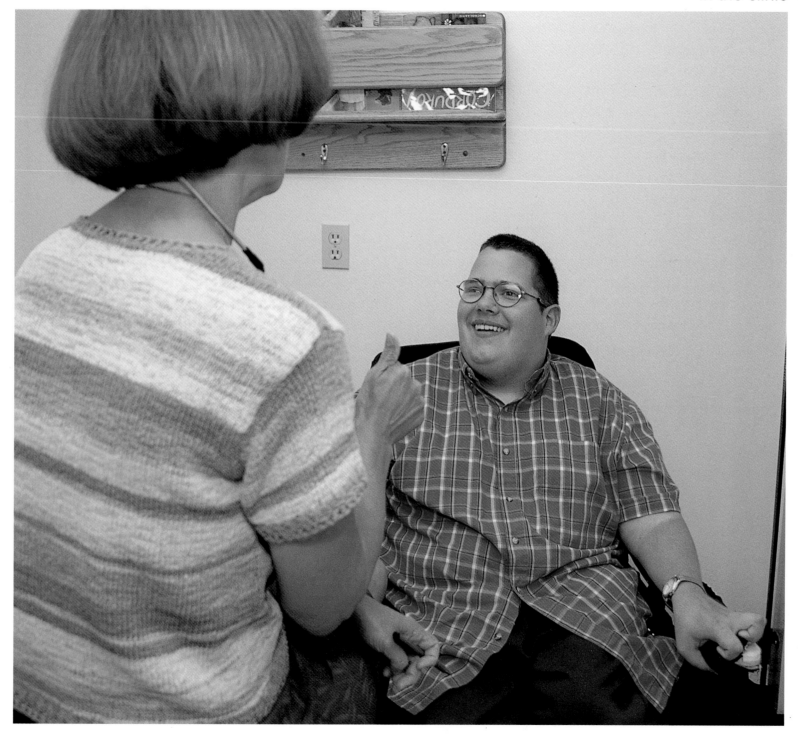

lems due to a childhood of abuse. In his smoldering anger, he had kicked a chair that day and injured his foot. She slowly squeezed his toes, working on up to his ankle. Since there was no pain reaction and she saw no swelling, he didn't need an Xray. She advised him to take a pain killer and, more important, to be sure to continue with his Prozac to prevent such tumultuous eruptions.

Before seeing her next patient, Phyllis was interrupted by a call from another doctor. It's an unwritten rule that physicians answer each other's phone calls immediately. However, this call was somewhat irritating, since it wasn't about a patient, but rather a new HMO contract that had just been mailed out. The business of medicine was continuing to insinuate itself into the practice of healing.

... another asthmatic

Patient 19 had lost his asthma inhaler a year ago and now was in some respiratory panic because of cough. As Phyllis listened to his chest, she heard no wheezing, however. While she reassured him and prescribed a new inhaler, she also preached to him what she called rule number one for asthmatics: "Never be without your inhaler."

... a sore throat

As she did many times a day, Phyllis had to convince the mother of **patient 20**, an 11-year-old girl, that her daughter's sore throat was caused by a virus and didn't need antibiotics.

... is there pus in the hip?

An 8-year-old girl, **patient 21**, complained of sudden pain in her hip. Phyllis felt fairly sure that it was just a sprain. But in the back of the pediatrician's mind, the questions bubbled forth: "Is there something else going on? Is some disease just starting? Is there infection with pus in the joint? Is the head of the hip bone beginning to slip off?" Making even the simplest of diagnoses can often be a worry for a pediatrician. If the diagnosis is missed, it may become a nightmare for the patient and a malpractice suit for the doctor.

Phyllis picked up the child's leg at the ankle and knee and bent her hip forward; there was no grimace of pain. She moved the bent knee, first to the inside and then outwardly: there was no cry. She instructed the girl to walk; there was no limping.

Phyllis once again convinced herself that this just had to be a sprain, and that she didn't need to put the child through a hospitalization, needle aspiration of the hip joint, and IV antibiotics. Yet the nagging question of pus in the hip still lurked. So she instructed her mother to bring the girl back if the pain persisted.

... is it leukemia?

Patient 22, a 2-year-old, was a real worry. She had been seen a day earlier in the Emergency Department with a fever of 103 to 105 following an illness that had stretched out for two weeks. Though a blood test came back suggesting that it was just a viral illness, there was a slight hint from the high

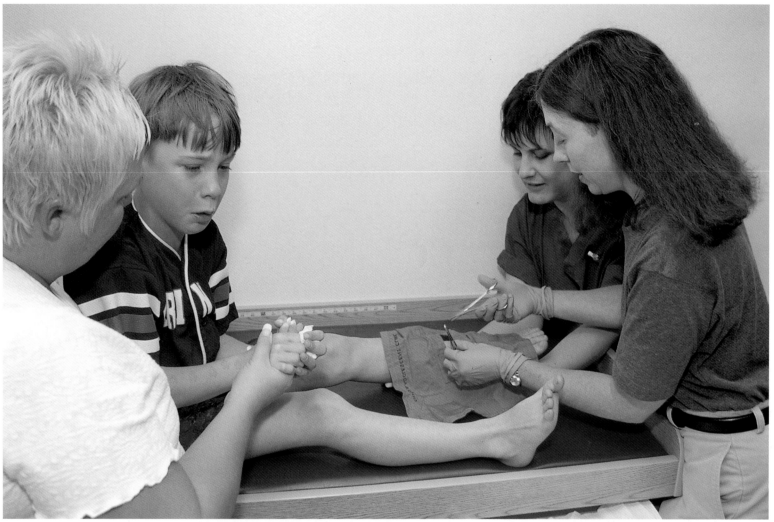

Any clinic day can be interrupted by an emergency laceration. Krystopher Grubbs had cut his leg. With the comforting support of his mother, he is able to control his anxiety as Dr. Sue Abell, right, and nurse Trudy Custer repair his laceration. (After Dr. Abell finished suturing, Krystopher expressed surprise that it really didn't hurt. Trudy had applied a topical anesthetic with a gauze pad before the minor surgery started, avoiding the use of a scary needle)

lymphocyte count and low platelets that this could be leukemia.

Phyllis's heart sank. She knew she was going to have to handle this and tell the parent that there was a very slight possibility of cancer, and that another blood test was needed. She also was fully aware from past experience that at the very mention of the word "leukemia," parents' emotions sink so far through the floor that they hear little more of what is said. Nevertheless, she had no choice but to inform the mother of these tentative findings.

The mother remained stoic as the doctor told her that a blood smear needed to be sent to the pathologist for his reading. That takes time. It was undoubtedly a sleepless night for the parents, but the next day Phyllis was joyous to report to them that the test was normal. No leukemia.

... rule out dehydration

The last visit, **patient 23**, was a 2-year-old boy with vomiting and diarrhea. Since there was no blood in the stool, the most likely cause was a viral infection. Phyllis checked the child's oral membranes and skin, finding no obvious dehydration. But little ones can dry out quickly, so she gave his mother instructions on pushing salt and sugar fluids into the child to prevent it.

... caring with paperwork

Leaving this last patient of the day, Dr. Phyllis Cavens slumped into her desk chair. Since she had started clinic after hospital rounds an hour later than usual, she hadn't seen her usual thirty patients that day, but she was tired.

Before her was a mound of charts yet to be reviewed. Consult letters from other doctors had to be read. Letters had to be dictated to agencies to get services for some of the patients. Phone calls had to be returned. Though this is derisively called "paperwork," Phyllis in her more generous, reflective moments realizes that this extra hour or two of work is a time when she helps shape the lives of children forever by being their advocate.

Being an advocate for children doesn't always help, however. For years most pediatricians have tried to dissuade the practice of infant circumcision, but to little avail.

Circumcision

It hurts. For centuries, humankind has preferred to pretend that circumcising the male infant is relatively painless. For decades, pediatricians have felt a twinge of concern as they crushed a narrow wedge of foreskin with forceps to begin the procedure.

They wondered: Did infants really feel less pain as they had been taught? If so, why was the baby crying? Was it just because he was being held down?

No one knew the answers for sure, but with recent laboratory studies, we now know that male infants do feel it. It has been shown that they have less discomfort if they have some form of pain control. If a local anesthetic is injected into the penis, crying and fast heart rates are decreased about 50 percent on an average. In addition, blood levels of cortisol are lower, indicating that the baby is suffering less stress.

Relieving such distress begs the bigger question, however. Should infants be circumcised at all? There is very little rea-

Opposite: After injecting an anesthetic in the baby's penis, Dr. Blaine Tolby cuts the foreskin prior to removing it.

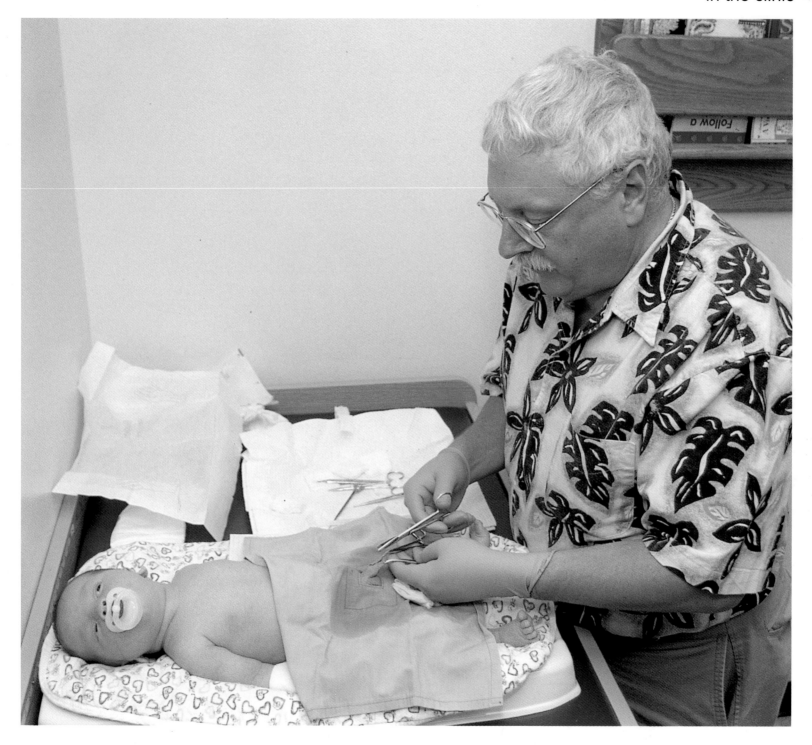

son to do it for health purposes. The American Academy of Pediatrics has proclaimed that in spite of some potential medical benefits, "the data are not sufficient to recommend routine neonatal circumcision."

Rather than being a medical necessity, circumcision is more a custom in the United States. It is uncommon in Asia, South America, Central America, and most of Europe. During World War II, the Germans used circumcision as a way of identifying Jewish people or U.S. spies.

The procedure gained acceptance in the U.S. due to several factors, foremost being our Judeo-Christian heritage. The Hebrew males that Moses led out of Egypt underwent circumcision, following the example of their Egyptian masters (whose mummies disclose the practice). Men who visited the Hebrews could not participate in the Passover unless they and their male servants were circumcised (Exodus 12:48).

Centuries later, the tradition of circumcision proved to be a stumbling block to Greeks and Romans, whom the apostle Paul was trying to convert to Christianity; they weren't too enthusiastic about that part of the new religion. At the Council of Jerusalem in 49 A.D., Paul was able to convince the elders after much arguing that circumcision wasn't a necessary requirement (Acts 15:1-12).

Nevertheless, the Old Testament teaching held fast in this country. This was coupled with the observation during World War I that men fighting in the trenches, unable to keep clean, sometimes developed an infection of the penis. This gave support to the idea that it would be better to circumcise in infancy as a preventive.

And so, circumcision is a procedure ingrained in our culture that pediatricians reluctantly perform, but strive to do as kindly as possible.

"Lucky Baby"

They waited anxiously in a hotel room in China. Finally LeeAnn and Ted McLean were filled with wonder as the agency representative handed them their 11-month-old baby. She was a girl, as almost all the adopted babies are in China. They named her "Asia" — Asia McLean.

During their walks on the city streets, they were frequently surprised when Chinese strangers approached them to declare in understandable English, "Lucky baby."

And indeed Asia was lucky. Her alert expression and rounded body gave assurances that she had received loving care by her Chinese foster mother. Still, there were questions about her health and development; therefore, her new parents brought her to the pediatrician the day after they arrived back in the United States.

Phyllis examined her carefully. She ordered blood tests for anemia, syphilis and hepatitis, plus a stool sample to be sent to the lab to test for parasites. Asia's immunization record and tuberculosis tests were reviewed. Phyllis then assured Ted and LeeAnn that their new baby was quite normal and that she would be helping them with Asia's adaptation to her new "niche."

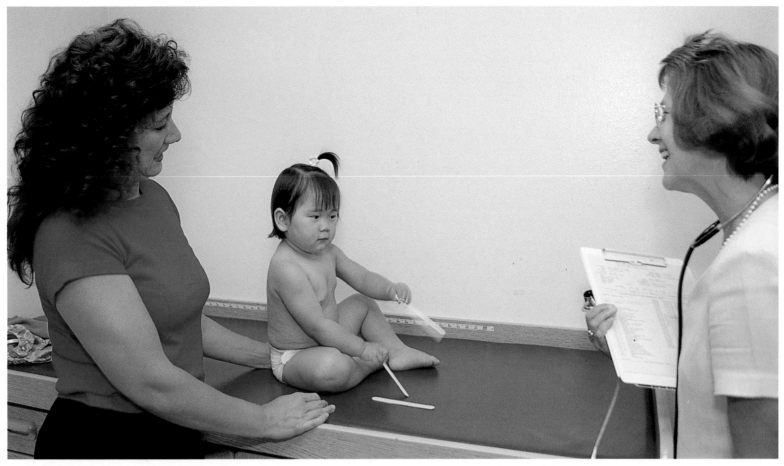

Twenty-two-month-old Asia McLean shows off her "drum roll" to Phyllis who is pleased to observe this demonstration of good intellectual development. Asia was adopted by LeeAnn (above left) and Ted McLean at 11 months of age.

"Niche" is a new term that is being embraced by pediatricians that refers to the social setting. A child's destiny is no longer considered merely a conflict between "nature" vs. "nurture," but rather, a dynamic relationship between all three elements — nature plus nurture plus niche. Asia brought with her the genes she had been dealt (nature); LeeAnn and Ted were to provide a new loving environment (nurture); and together they would interact within the environment of family,

friends, community and doctor (the niche). The niche, therefore, is a link between parents and offspring, an envelope of life chances. Asia's chances appeared so rich.

As LeeAnn and Ted were boarding the plane with Asia at the airport in China, their excitement was tempered by a scene of sadness. There were four other happy couples in line with them, each with a Chinese baby girl. But standing silently far away from the group were two people, a Chinese man and woman, whose eyes followed one of the babies as the Americans filed out. Their baby was leaving on that plane forever. Their expression of grief suggested a pain as great as if death had visited them.

Death Is a Stranger

Pediatricians rarely deal with death. Most of them, if asked, could sit down and recall all the children they cared for that passed away. They would remember little ones who died suddenly of gunshots, auto accidents or meningococcemia, or patients who struggled longer with leukemia or incurable malformations. But it would not be a long list, since death is a relative stranger to pediatricians.

Unlike other kinds of doctors who treat adults and face death more frequently, pediatricians are not accustomed to such occurences. They may, therefore, allow themselves to get closer to their patients, but risk being more emotionally affected when one does die.

They may have some desire to attend the funeral of a stricken child, but are hesitant to do so, feeling that in some way they have failed — a child is dead. Phyllis, however, has been welcomed at funerals of patients and found it to be personally soothing, not only to the family, but to her, too.

While the death of most children is remembered well, there is one type of child who dies largely unknown. It is the stillborn baby who never had a chance to interact and develop a personality. That baby never established an identity with most people except, for two important individuals — the baby's parents, especially the mother. To her, the baby was a person. It moved. It reacted to light and sound. She talked to her baby. The mother's pain of losing such a one has been compared to an amputation — the loss of an arm or leg.

Well-meaning friends will try to console her by saying, "You'll get over it. You'll have another baby." They don't understand, however, the nature of the mother-baby bond that existed. The pediatrician's job is to acknowledge the mother's grief, educating those around her as to its intensity.

Bonding to Twins

The premature delivery of Julie and Rick Garcia's twins upset their carefully laid plans of opening a restaurant in Denver. Their babies were supposed to be born in that city after they moved from Longview. But birth came earlier than expected, with Andrew weighing 3 pounds, 2 ounces and Ali 2 pounds, 11 ounces. The two were immediately transferred to Doernbecher Children's Hospital in Portland, Oregon, for a two-month stay.

Mr. and Mrs. Garcia didn't give up their dream, however, of moving to Colorado. Shortly after their babies were discharged from the hospital, they decided to make that move. Even though Andrew still required oxygen, Phyllis felt they could make the journey.

The highway patrol was alerted in each state. Rick and Julie hired a nurse from Doernbecher's neonatal unit to travel with them in the car, checking oxygen levels as they drove over the mountain passes. (The airlines had declined to fly them.) Both babies arrived safely.

Months later, Julie visited her family in Longview. Her boy, Andrew, suffered from chronic congestion and prior remedies had not worked. She, therefore, brought him to see Phyllis for a trusted second opinion. Phyllis switched him to a soybean formula that proved successful.

Twins, of course, are fascinating. Because they are less common, occurring only once in every 88 pregnancies, family members and friends often exhibit behavior that is unusual in regards to newborns. First, they carefully scrutinize both of the babies to see how much they look alike. And next, they give them "twin" gifts, clothes that are identical.

There is a psychological reason given for this. People would rather think of twins as one. They want the babies to be as much alike as possible, because it is easier to bond to one human at a time rather than two. (The same principle is in effect when an adult falls in love; they are "head-over-heels in love" with one person and not a group.)

Thus, when two individuals are born of the same mother at the same time, they are often considered "the twins" — a single unit — rather than two babies with identifying first names.

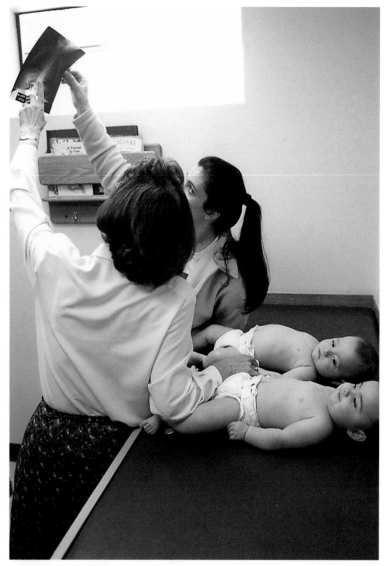

Julie Garcia is reassured that the chest Xray of 8-month-old Andrew is normal.

It is the pediatrician's job to advise the family to treat each child as an individual by dressing them differently, arranging unique activities for each, placing them in different classes in school and, of course, using their first names.

The Garcias have followed through with this advice, making sure that their two babies are known as Ari and Andrew, separate persons. As their father Rick points out, however, it is a little easier since they are a boy and a girl.

4 ... on call

Availability to patients, day or night, is a duty that most doctors in private practice feel is part of their medical responsibility. But the task has become more onerous over the past decades as technology, which should make things easier, has actually made life tougher.

In bygone ages, doctors couldn't be reached so easily. If there was a medical emergency on the farm, it was often necessary for a relative to get on a horse and ride into town to get "Doc." Since it wasn't an easy thing to do, it wasn't done very often. But this was an era before phones and their dreadful descendants, pagers, whose appearance changed the lives of doctors forever.

Pediatricians especially are beleaguered by easy accessibility. After the office closes, they may try to carry on with their normal family events, but the phone will ring a completely unpredictable number of times. Sometimes there will be a dozen calls, extending through the dinner and evening hours and on through the night. And sometimes — very rarely — it won't ring at all, giving the doctor an uneasy feeling that something has gone terribly wrong with the system, and that some child may be dying because they have failed to respond.

The phone often rings at inopportune times. It will interrupt just as the family sits down for dinner or during the last five minutes of the dramatic conclusion of the TV movie of

Phyllis awakens instantly when the phone rings in the middle of the night in order to give accurate advice.

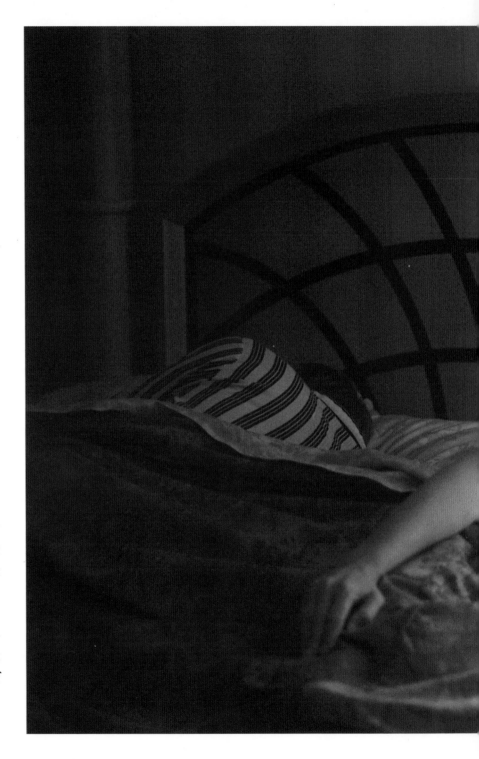

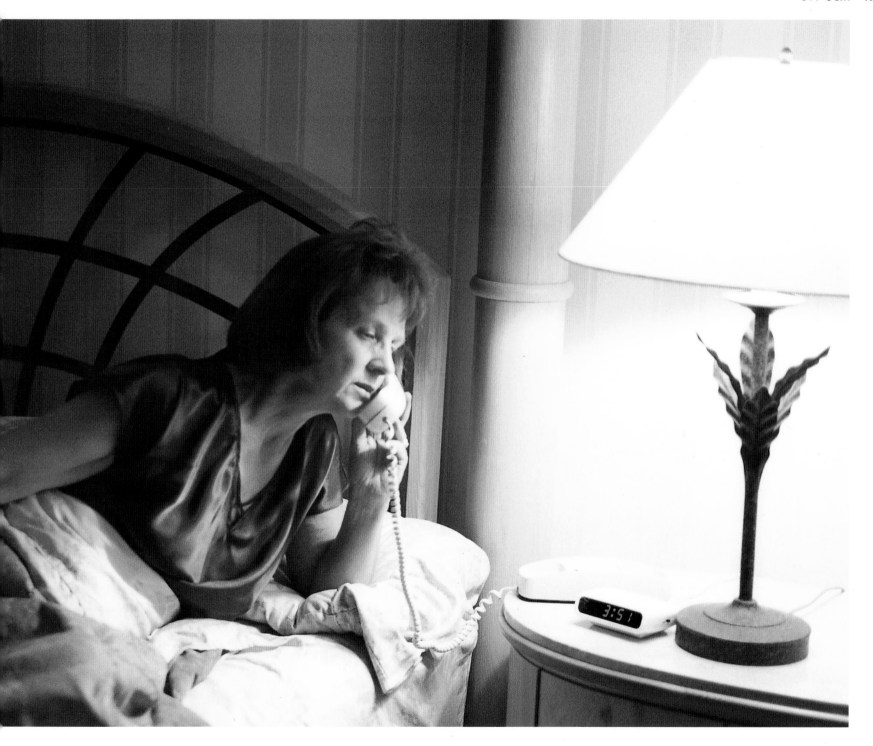

the week. And if the parent who is calling hears the doctor breathing hard, it may not be because of a quick run to the phone, but rather due to a maddening pause in making love.

Trading Call

One of the main reasons that doctors form partnerships is to trade call, so that they can get nights and weekends away from the incessant phone or pager. If there are two physicians working together, each of them can get away half the time and, of course, if there are more physicians in the group, they can all have more free time.

But there is a catch. The more doctors there are in a medical group, the more patients there are to care for, and that might be overwhelming for the partner whose turn it is to cover. The pace can be exhausting due to long hours, worry and lack of sleep.

When the physician finishes such a rotation and recovers in a day or so, he or she can cheerfully look forward to weeks of relative calm. They made it through the ordeal, and so they can relax for a while. But as the time of the month approaches when they are once again to go on call, irritation and impatience begin to mount, somewhat analogous to PMS.

Some phone calls are thoughtless such as, "My child has a toothache and I didn't want to wake our dentist." But all the calls from parents, frivolous or not, reflect worry about their youngster. They may phone from a hotel room in a distant city because their child has developed a fever during the family vacation. Being in a strange place, they are frantic and need

to hear a trusted voice, giving words of assurance and decision.

Rushing to the Hospital

When a parent calls at night, Phyllis must snap awake in order to sort out a minor problem from serious disease. Questions need to be asked about fever and the child's ability to respond. She needs to know if there is a rash and, if so, what it looks like. If the answer is that the baby has purple-colored spots, a picture of the dreaded disease meningococcemia rushes through her mind. The parent catches the ex-

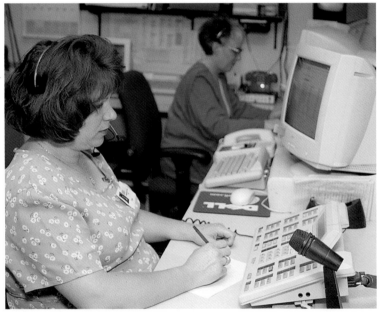

Tammy Miller and Bonnie King are paging operators hidden away in the basement of St. John Medical Center where they are never seen. Each is a disembodied voice — a very familiar but faceless voice that beckons physicians to awaken and respond to the newest emergency.

treme anxiety in her voice as she urges them to rush the child to the emergency room.

As Phyllis hangs up, she immediately redials the hospital to bark out stat orders to the nurse to prepare for the child's arrival. Her clothes have been laid out, ready to be pulled on. She runs to open the garage door to begin the race to the ER.

If it is late at night and traffic is light, Phyllis may gamble with her own safety as she speeds through empty intersections against red lights. She counts on the fact that the police in the town know her car and will escort her on, if they do happen to spot her.

In similar nighttime phone calls, the doctor's heart also races when awakened by the nurse working on labor and delivery with the message that the obstetrician needs a pediatrician "to come right in." This almost always means that a baby is in trouble during the birth process.

The same type of mad rush to the hospital ensues. After the delivery, the mother's doctor may be able to go home soon, but Phyllis is often in for a high-intensity night, treating a baby with infection or respiratory distress. And so the phone often brings dreaded news out of the blue.

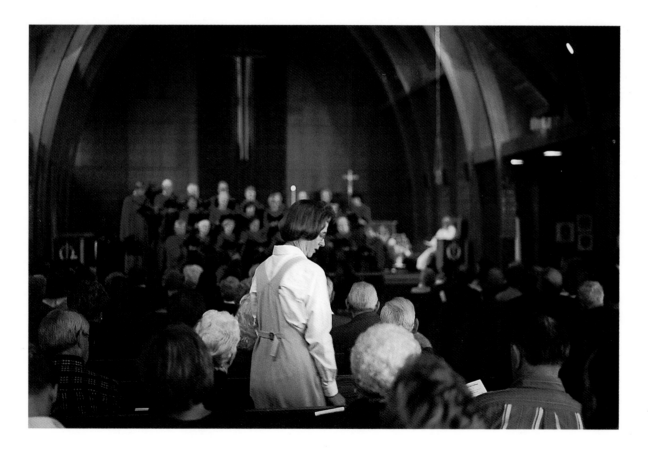

Phyllis leaves in the middle of the Sunday service at Emmanuel Lutheran Church after being paged. Any pediatrician who answers phone calls from parents on weekends or nights is often interrupted in church, at the movies or during their children's soccer games.

5 ... *keeping up*

It Starts in Medical School

The anxiety starts the first time the freshman medical student lifts the required textbooks about human anatomy, physiology and biochemistry from the bookstore counter. Each is two to three inches thick, weighing multiple pounds. The student knows that these are not just reference books in which to access arcane facts, but that those tomes contain volumes of material that is to be studied and understood.

Indeed, that initial anxiety — that pressure that begins on the first day of medical school — never lets up. There is always the fear that some fact, unknown to the physician and not acted on, could lead to a patient's death or a colleague's derision — or a lawsuit.

A lifelong struggle ensues between an internal guilt-laden voice that says you are not spending enough time reading the medical literature, versus those external forces that call for pursuing other interests, either alone or with family and friends, that may be just plain fun.

There are times, however, when a doctor can do both: learn as well as relax. There are periodic events where one can get away from the frantic pace of practice, meet old friends, eat leisurely romantic dinners and still keep up with what is new in pediatrics. These events are the professional conferences held in nearby medical centers or in intriguing cities throughout the world.

The National AAP Conference

The grande dame of pediatric conferences is the American Academy of Pediatrics annual meeting. It is big. It is glitzy and exciting. More than ten thousand pediatricians gather from all over the U.S. and the world to learn and to be revitalized.

There is usually an inspirational keynote speaker who reminds the physicians that they belong to a profession devoted to the healing of children. One year, the pediatricians jumped to their feet with tears in their eyes at the end of a cozy, warm talk by Fred ("Mr.") Rogers, who touched their very being as doctors of little boys and girls. At another time, retired U.S. Army Gen. Colin Powell showed his strong father image, as he laid out dreams for America's children, once again bringing the audience to its feet.

... the teaching at the AAP meeting

But for those AAP delegates who want more detail and desire specific knowledge, there are more than 130 seminars, workshops, and short talks from which to select. Topics vary yearly and range from "Basic EKG Interpretation" to "The Child with Cough" to "Pelvic Exam."

Right: A squadron of buses transports pediatricians from the hotels of San Francisco to the Moscone Convention Center during the 1998 AAP fall meeting.

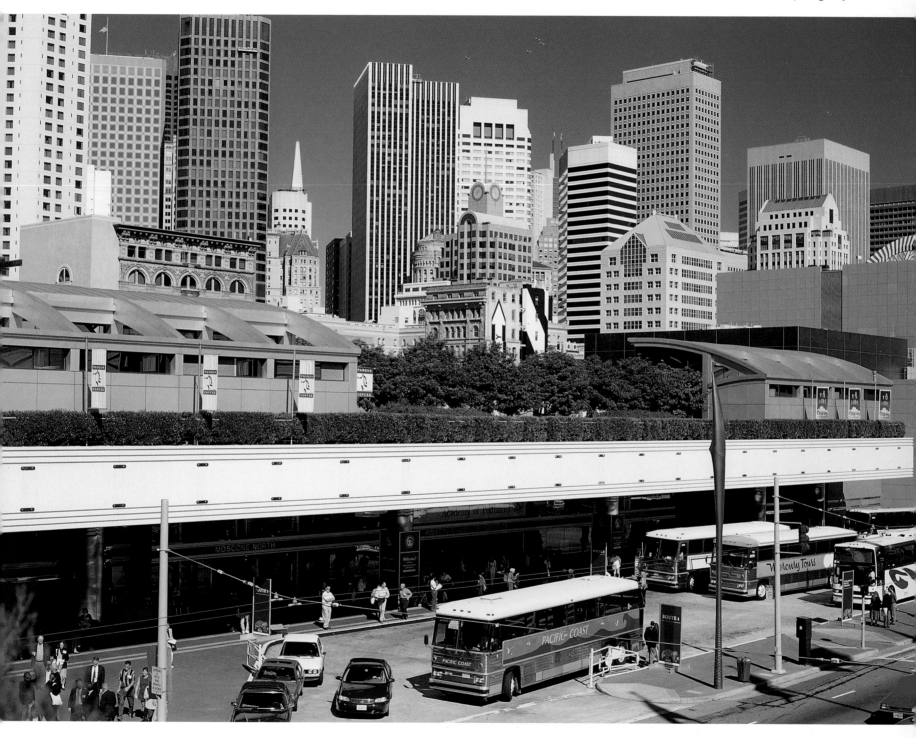

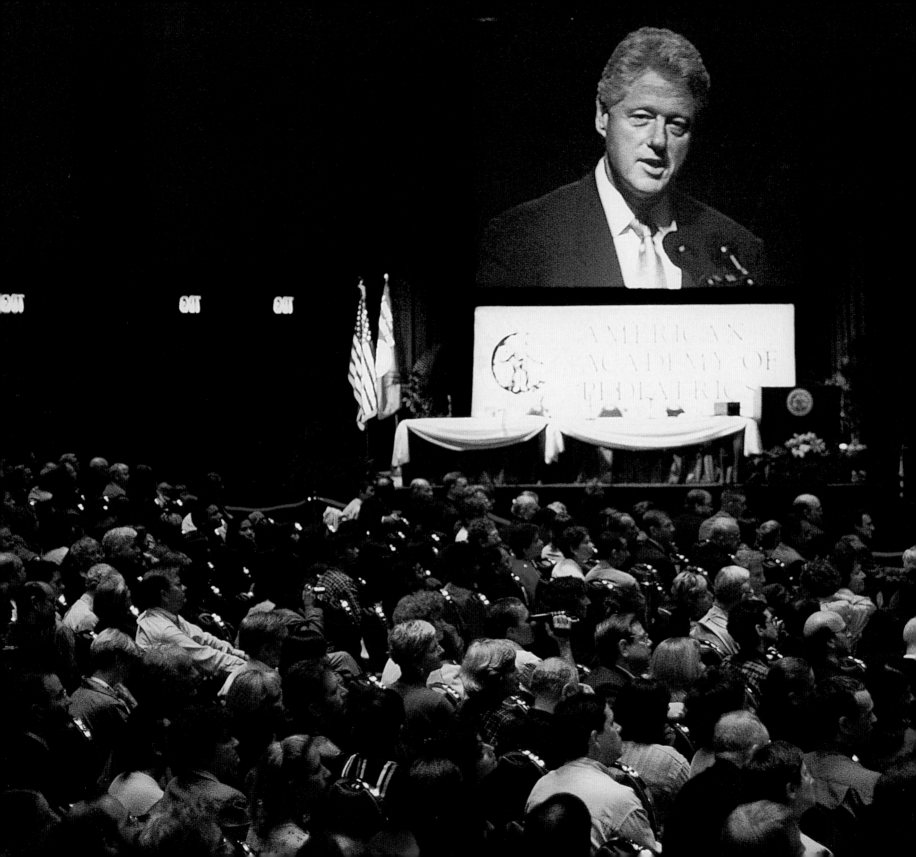

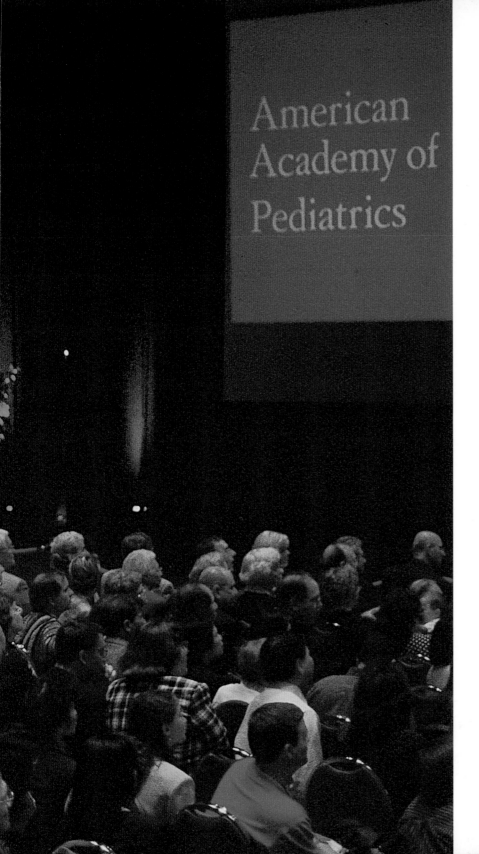

... the Red Book Committee

One presentation at the AAP conference, called "Meeting the Red Book Committee," has become an unchanging tradition. The Red Book is the bible of pediatrics, giving the most current recommendations on the treatment of infectious disease. And since infectious disease is the bread and butter of pediatric practice, pediatricians are intensely interested in what those committee members who write the book have to say.

Microphones are planted in the aisles. The doctors line up so that, one by one, they can ask the experts for their opinions on new vaccines and antibiotics. Usually, there is a questioner or two from another country, and one realizes that this is indeed an international meeting.

... the passion of pediatricians

Pediatricians take pride in their organization, the AAP, since its main purpose is to provide the best medical care for children. Very little discussion takes place on improving personal incomes or working conditions of doctors.

Phyllis saw two of her old friends at the 1998 meeting who exemplified the passion that most pediatricians have for improving the lot of all children. For instance, Dr. Allen Harlor, chairperson of the AAP Council on Governmental Affairs, reported on three initiatives to help children that the AAP had tried to present to the U.S. Congress. His voice

The image of Bill Clinton, president of the United States, is projected overhead as he speaks in person to several thousand pediatricians at the 1999 AAP conference in Washington, D.C.

cracked with emotion as he explained that their efforts had been in vain because Congressional members were too busy fighting among themselves.

At another meeting, Dr. Gerda Benda scurried across the meeting hall to get her written suggestion to the chairman, refusing to have it ignored.   She was proposing that the 10,000 pediatricians who would have gathered at the next meeting in Washington D.C. should march on the capital on behalf of children.

Her proposal wasn't accepted, but it exemplifies the concern that the 55,000 members of the American Academy of Pediatrics have for the young of America. Committees continually work on diverse childhood issues such as nicotine addiction, access to medical care, immunizations, day care, and many more.

Supporting these issues helps bond the delegates and makes them aware that they are not alone in their struggles for children. So much of their practices back home consists of confrontational dealings with insurance carriers, hospitals and other medical specialists, but here, in the comradeship of other pediatricians, they develop resolve.

More than 300 exhibitors crowd the floor of the Washington Conference Center during the 1999 annual AAP meeting.

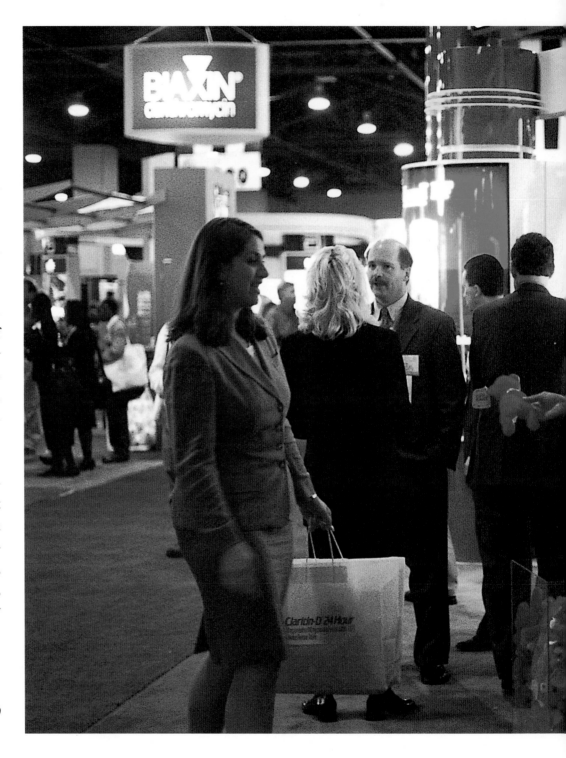

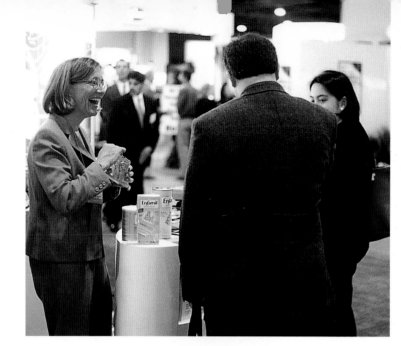

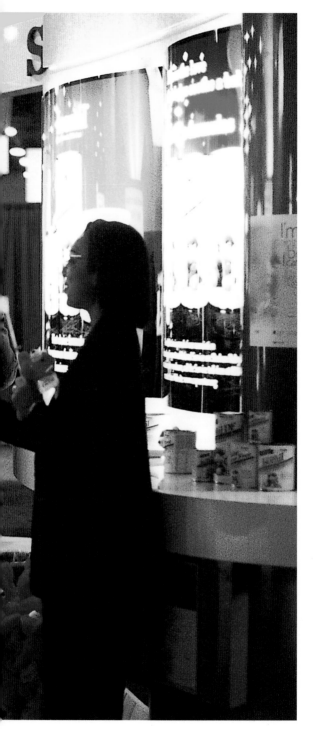

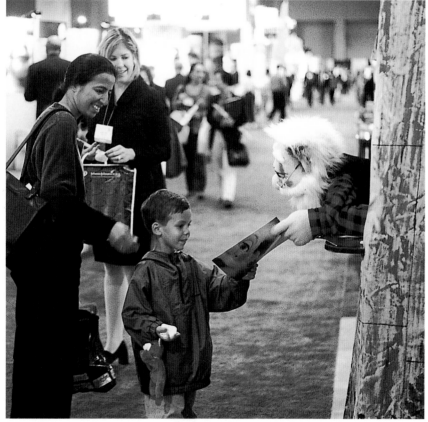

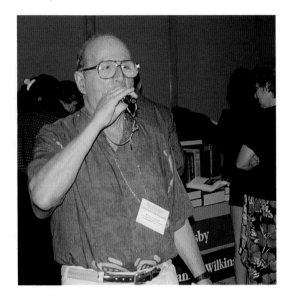

Above: Using his celebrated duck call, Dr. Milton Arnold calls pediatricians back to the lecture room after the midmorning "fluids in - fluids out" break of the 1999 Combined Southern California Pediatric Postgraduate Meeting in Palm Springs.

Regional Conferences

Besides the national conferences, there are smaller meetings held throughout the United States where pediatricians can learn what is new and also earn CME (Continuing Medical Education) credits to maintain their state license to practice. These teaching sessions often take place at medical schools, but also are put on at destination resorts.

The AAP's California District Nine and Chapter 2, jointly organize conferences in Las Vegas, Hawaii, Tahoe, and Palm Springs. Those meetings have been successful largely through the thirty years of work by its scientific programs chairman, Dr. Milton Arnold, who shows that a doctor in general pediatric practice can be a strong voice in medical education.

Right: Phyllis sits between two friends she has made over the years while attending the Palm Springs conference, David and Venny Knoop from Mendham, New Jersey.

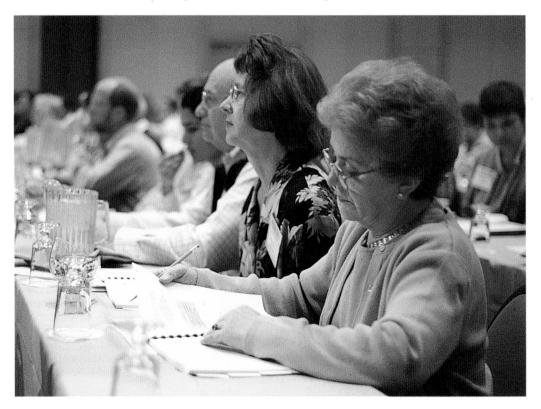

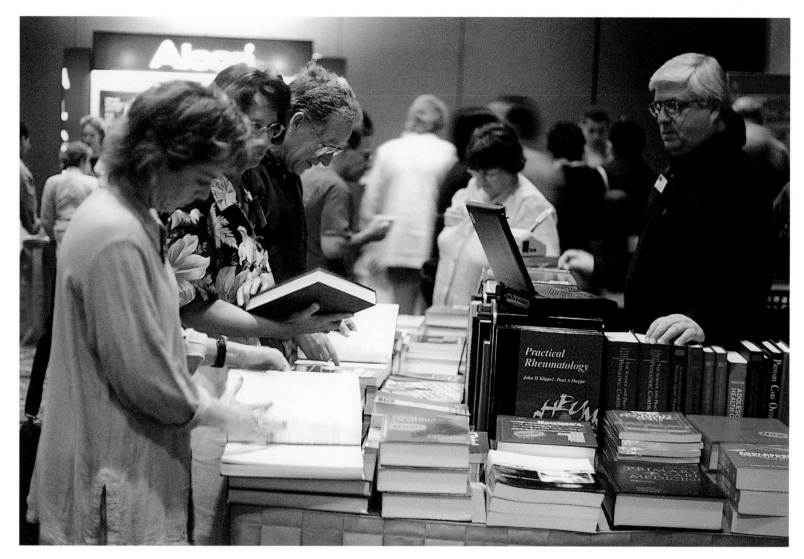

Pediatricians pore through the latest books for sale during a break at the 1999 Palm Springs conference, feeling a need to update their office libraries despite the steep cost of medical texts. For instance, the venerable classic Nelson Textbook of Pediatrics *now sells for one hundred and ten dollars. (The text was first compiled by Dr. Waldo E. Nelson in 1933, and the work is now in its sixteenth edition. It is said that Dr. Nelson's daughter helped in the tedious task of writing the index, and that she slipped in "Pediatrics - for the birds.")*

Training for the Emergency

At every pediatric clinic, there is a chance that a potential disaster may come screaming through its doors at any time. A child may be rushed in, pale, stuporous, and gasping for air. Death may be minutes away.

The well-run office is prepared. Oxygen and IV fluids are on hand, and the nursing staff are trained to get all the equipment and materials needed stat. But the pressure still falls on the pediatrician to make an instant evaluation of the child and to act.

This requires training and practice. Many physicians, along with nurses, repeatedly take a course called PALS or Pediat-ric Advanced Life Support, which is offered by key children's hospitals throughout the country.

The primary aim of the course is to review new information about resuscitation and to practice giving lifesaving treatment to a child, even before a diagnosis is knowable.

Prior to 1978, there were no standardized techniques for the resuscitation of children. Earlier, the American Heart Association had developed emergency care for adults, but eventually it became evident that young people didn't die of adult diseases such as heart attacks or strokes. The AHA, therefore, initiated the development of emergency care standards for children, which in turn led to the PALS course.

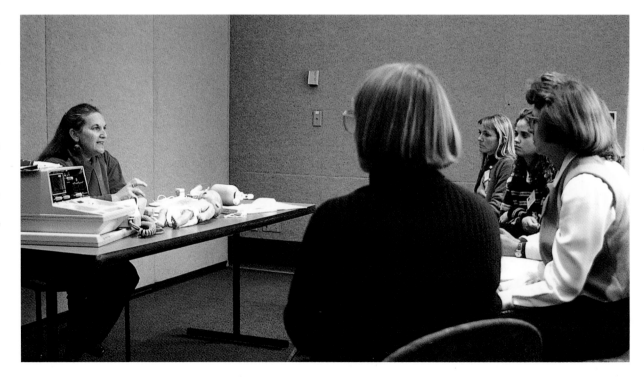

At a PALS course in Portland, Oregon, neonatal nurse Gina Craven stresses that, unlike in adults, there are only three abnormal heart rates in children that pediatricians really have to know: fast, slow — or none.

17:17-22. Elijah took a child from its mother's arms whose "illness was so severe that there was no breath left in him." He laid him on a bed and "stretched himself upon the child three times" so that "the life of the child came into him again, and he revived."

It can be assumed that Elijah was very excited while performing this procedure for he "...cried to the Lord...." His heart and breathing rates were probably racing just like anyone resuscitating a child today. During the PALS course, doctors feel similar stress while doing mock resuscitation even though there are no real patients.

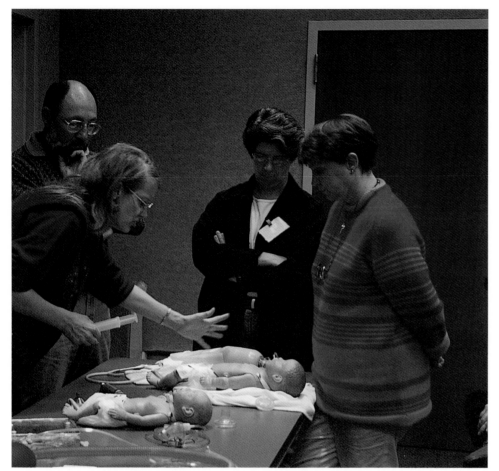

With her usual whirlwind exuberance, Dr. Cindy Cristofani makes a lifesaving point during a megacode practice. Dr. Cristofani has championed the PALS course at Legacy Emanuel Children's Hospital in Portland, Oregon, for more than a decade.

... each worries about their response

The instructors of the PALS course have developed "megacodes" that simulate emergency situations of patients. The students (doctors and nurses) are expected to respond quickly to these megacodes. In a typical teaching situation, they are asked to gather around a table that is strewn with mannequins, tubes, and oxygen bags, plus an electronic monitor that can exhibit different heart problems at the flick of a switch.

The students are then read an opening scene in which a child comes into the emergency room in desperate straits, and the question is thrown at them, "What do you do first?" They may ask for lab data, which may or not be available.

... recorded in the Old Testament

An instruction manual was composed for the PALS course, but the authors humbly admit that they were not the first to write about pediatric resuscitation. A lifesaving event was recorded in the Old Testament 2,800 years ago, in 1 Kings

They may order a medicine, and the instructor may say the "patient" did improve but now is disintegrating with a falling oxygen level. "What's happening?"

Even though everyone knows this is all a mock exercise, and even though the instructors have said that they don't intend to flunk anyone, there is tension. The students are all putting their intelligence out for everyone to see, something they haven't done since school.

The doctors are worried about the nurses looking smarter than they (which they may be); the new students are concerned that they don't have any experience; and the older practitioners see bright, young people moving in on them. In the mind of each of them, however, lurks that fear that they won't be able to respond properly in an actual situation, and so they work hard at relearning.

... hesitant to cut

Besides rehearsing megacodes, the students also practice doing hands-on surgical procedures, such as inserting a large tube through the chest wall into the lung cavity. Since pediatricians are not surgically minded and are hesitant by their nature to cut into the human body, many fear making such a decisive act. They realize, however, that a situation some day may force them to do it, and so they practice on the models set up.

Children in shock often need large volumes of fluid, but it may be impossible to get an intravenous line into their small, collapsed veins. An old technique has been rediscovered in which a large-bore needle is forced into the bone marrow of a small child, thereby obtaining lifesaving access to the blood stream. This interosseous technique is practiced on chicken legs, purchased at the grocery store. The "feel" of a large needle popping into the bone marrow of the chicken is very similar to that of inserting it into a 2-year-old.

... providing air — the art of intubation

Another technique that must be practiced over and over again is that of placing a tube for breathing into the trachea, which is much harder to do on a small child than it is on an adult. It is so easy to miss the child's trachea and place the tube unknowingly into the esophagus, a position that is useless. Or if the doctor is too excited, the tube can end up going down into the lung, or the laryngoscope blade can knock out teeth.

And so this technique, called intubation, is practiced repeatedly. Because this particular procedure is so important in providing air to a dying patient, students must be able to successfully do it during a timed test, or they will flunk the PALS course. They practice first on mannequins, but since these don't have the same characteristics as real people, cats sometimes are used.

These cats are loved and treated very tenderly. They are fully anesthetized, and the endotracheal tube is put down their throat with the same care as with any human undergoing surgery. The cats only have to go to "work" once a month, and at the end of two years, they retire from their "job" by being adopted out.

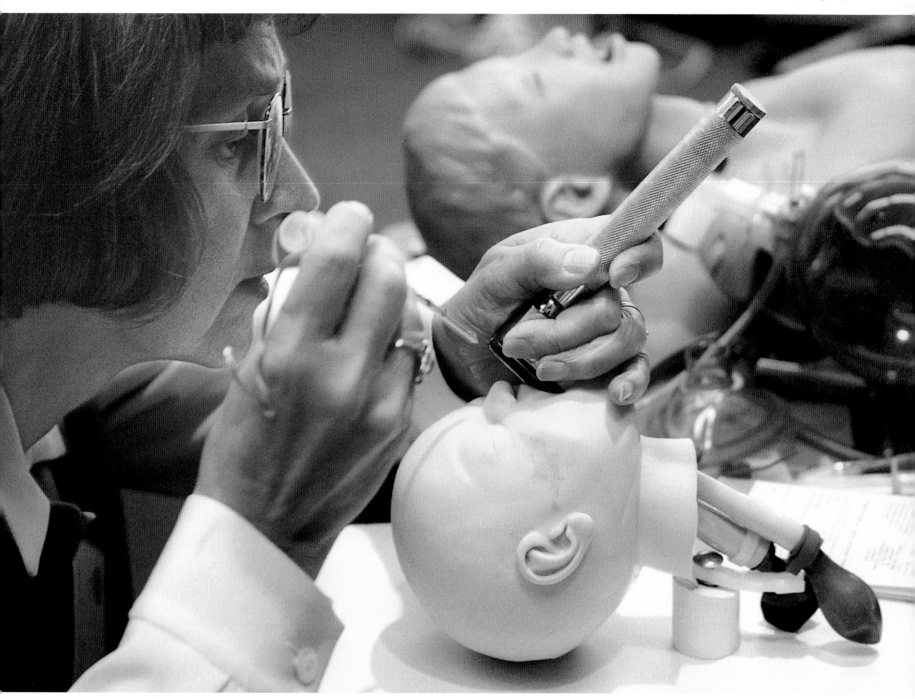

Phyllis practices lifting the laryngoscope blade to expose the glottis and slide a rubber tube down into the trachea of the mannequin.

6 ... in business

Competition in Medicine

Many doctors like to cling to the notion that they can practice medicine free of the unsavory aspects related to money. But there has always been a business side to medicine. Business is merely a tool by which service — good or bad — is given. As a service tool, it can be used either to provide quality medical care or curtail it; to introduce innovation or resist; to remain personal to patients or indifferent.

A decade ago, most doctors ran their own practices with simple business principles, similar to a "mom and pop grocery store." That suddenly changed as hospitals, insurance companies and HMOs formed large amalgamations. These corporations instituted controls that lessened inflation of health dollars (a positive step), but serious problems arose.

The public became concerned that unbridled managed care frequently denied them needed help or limited their choice of physician. Doctors in turn felt increased pressure to see more patients per day and to discharge them earlier from the hospital. Many physicians also experienced financial problems. They began to worry that they could not survive in the medical market place and sold their practices to for-profit medical corporations.

The partners of the Child and Adolescent Clinic decided to retain their independence and continue as private practitioners. They found themselves, however, competing not only with a large HMO, but also against their own local hospital, which had hired family doctors.

The clinic pediatricians countered by providing more services for their patients. They expanded their clinic hours to evenings and weekends, plus they added extra staff such as advice nurses and pediatric nurse practitioners.

Pediatric Nurse Practitioners

A few years ago, the pediatricians at the clinic employed a pediatric nurse practitioner. PNPs are registered nurses with an extra two years of training in pediatrics that qualifies them to diagnose and to prescribe medications. The use of a PNP was an experiment for the group at the time. The doctors had never worked with a nurse practitioner, and so they did not know what a PNP was capable of doing nor how patients would accept one.

Mary Dykes was the clinic's first pediatric nurse practitioner. She proved to be very competent, plus sought the doctors advice without hesitation whenever there was concern about a patient. More importantly, reports came back that parents were very pleased with her caring approach. Within months, two other PNPs, Mary Jane Hall and Pam Roberts, were added.

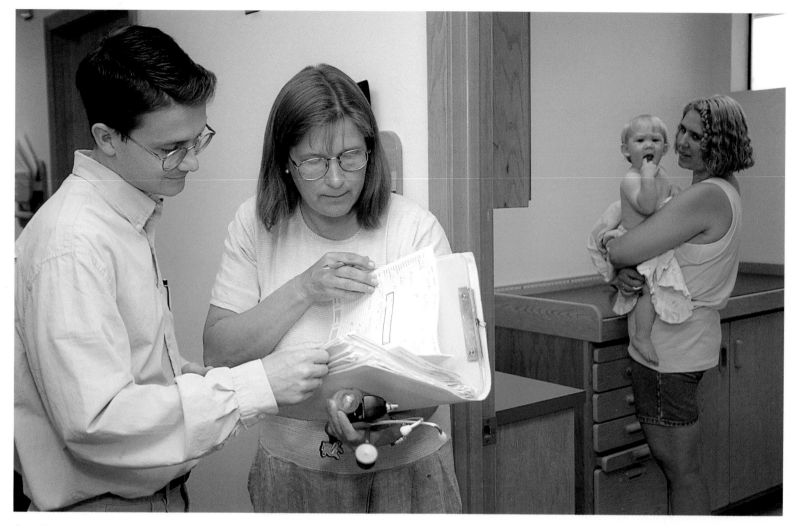

Dr. Aidan deRenne confers with Mary Dykes, a pediatric nurse practitioner, while patient Jonah Broderius and his mother wait quietly in the background.

Grow or Be Absorbed

As the practice expanded, the doctors once again debated how big their clinic should be. Their underlying philosophy was that they needed to grow to survive, but they worried that the cost of growth could be overwhelming.

Eventually, they determined that they had to be bigger. Two new doctors were added, as well as more examination rooms and office space. New computer and telephone systems were purchased, and an "Advice Nurse" position was created to answer the phone calls of concerned parents.

The doctors did hesitate, however, on making one major

business decision — to buy the empty land behind their clinic. They knew that the opportunity would soon disappear and along with it a chance to add more building and parking space in some distant future. It would be, however, a costly $290,000 venture, with the money to come from the personal finances of each partner. After many discussions, they agreed to buy it, knowing that they wouldn't really need it for years to come.

The question then arose as to what to do with the land in the meantime. There was some thought that they could pave it and rent out parking spaces, but the income would be rather small. Phyllis then had one of her novel ideas. Plant wildflowers and reap, instead of dollars, the pleasure of the beauty.

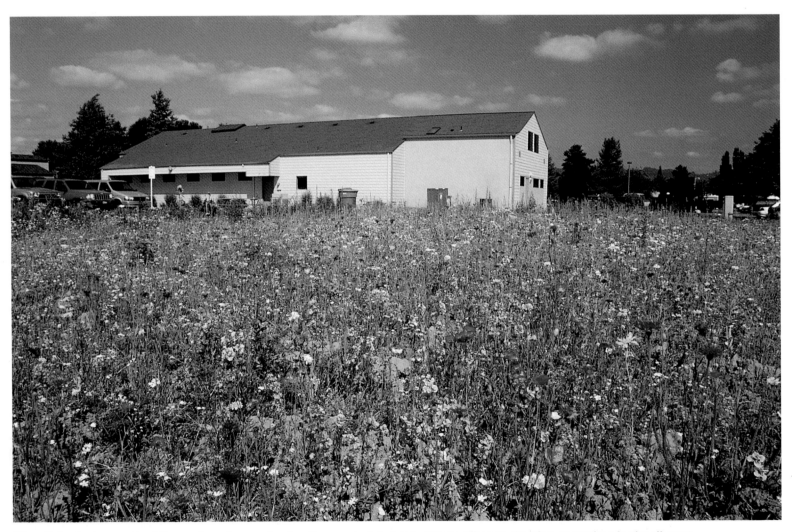

The clinic doctors extend themselves by purchasing the empty lots behind their office to develop sometime in the distant future. In the meantime, they plant wildflowers on the land.

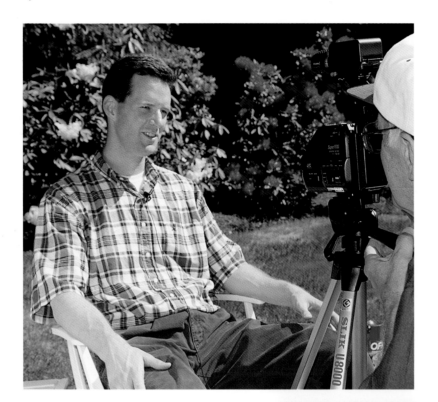

sign had to be less than three inches high, and the two-inch announcement in the newspaper could only run for one week. Display ads in the telephone book were unheard of.

That has all changed. The Child and Adolescent Clinic now has an outdoor sign that is lit up all night. An advertisement announcing a new pediatrician is in full color and takes up a half-page of the newspaper. The yellow pages ad in the telephone directory is no longer a few simple lines, but lists services and hours, and displays a picture of a pretty baby. In addition, the clinic has a Web page on the Internet and a monthly television program on community access TV.

Left: Dr. Randy Copeland is videotaped as he presents a lecture on preventing insect bites and rashes.

Below: John Glasco, the station manager of the community television station, KLTV, reviews Dr. Copeland's tape for broadcast.

Marketing the Practice

Competition has fostered a marked increase in advertising in the medical profession in recent years. Advertising (which doctors prefer to call "marketing") was not so blatant a few decades ago. Phyllis remembers a lecture given to members of her medical school class in the 1960s in which they were instructed on certain ethical advertising standards related to opening a practice. Their name on an outside

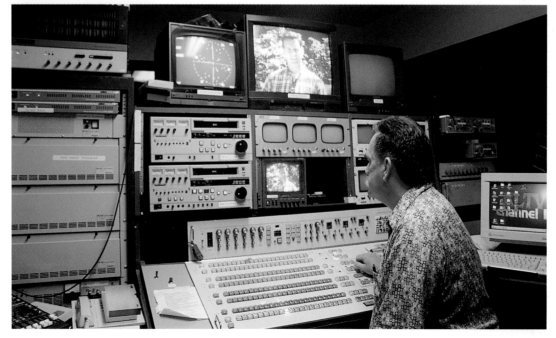

More importantly, however, there are strategy sessions where the doctors create ways to provide better medical care to their patients.

The Noon Meeting

To compete and expand takes a combined effort on the part of all the doctors of the clinic. Earlier in this book, I described the hectic day Phyllis had on December 17 (seeing a variety of patients). What was left out of that narrative was the weekly noon business meeting, sandwiched in between the morning and afternoon patients. That, too, was hectic.

On the agenda that particular noontime were twenty eight items. No one expected all of these to be dealt with in the scheduled one-and-a-half-hour meeting that was cut to one hour, but an attempt was made.

Dr. Blaine Tolby was already at his desk when Phyllis arrived. He was, in fact, lost in it. It was piled so high with charts and letters, the office staff couldn't find a landing place for phone messages; they piled them on his chair.

Dr. Kathleen Schatzel, who was wearing a splint for a recently fractured wrist, opened the meeting, but was interrupted by an emergency phone call; her daughter has been injured at school. She phoned her husband and asked him to go to the school to tend to Molly.

The meeting resumed with discussion of several major issues. "Should we buy the land behind the clinic?" "How do we handle the invitation to open a satellite office in St. Helens?" "When do we need to get new health insurance for the staff?" "How are we going to deal with the IPA?" All of these were major decisions. The business meeting finished late, as usual, with several partners trying to get in one more "must" item.

BUSINESS MEETING AGENDA

December 17, 12:30 to 2:00 p.m.

Expenses
　　Parking lot
　　St Helens clinic
　　Health insurance
　　PSI-IPA
　　Disability insurance
　　Health insurance
Marketing
　　Daily News ad
　　New OB
　　Patient satisfaction - waiting mom-toys/books
　　Pending video tapes
MD Schedule
　　On-call start time - 8 a.m.
　　MD call
Staff
　　Employee Assistance Program
Services
　　Hep A/Rotashield letter
　　Herbal medicine
　　Oral Polio #4
　　HIV testing CSA
　　Baby circular
　　Psych referrals
　　ADHD incentive papers
　　H21 hydrogen monitor
　　Foster kids and releasing information
　　Ped Dept meeting
　　Generic formula
　　OSHA conf
　　Old
　　U of W dental
　　Prenatal talks
　　Parents Place Newsletter

At the weekly business conference, all the doctors plus office manager Kimberly Robbins gather in the one room that is their office. The "no-walls" design promotes communication not only about business affairs, but also patient care.

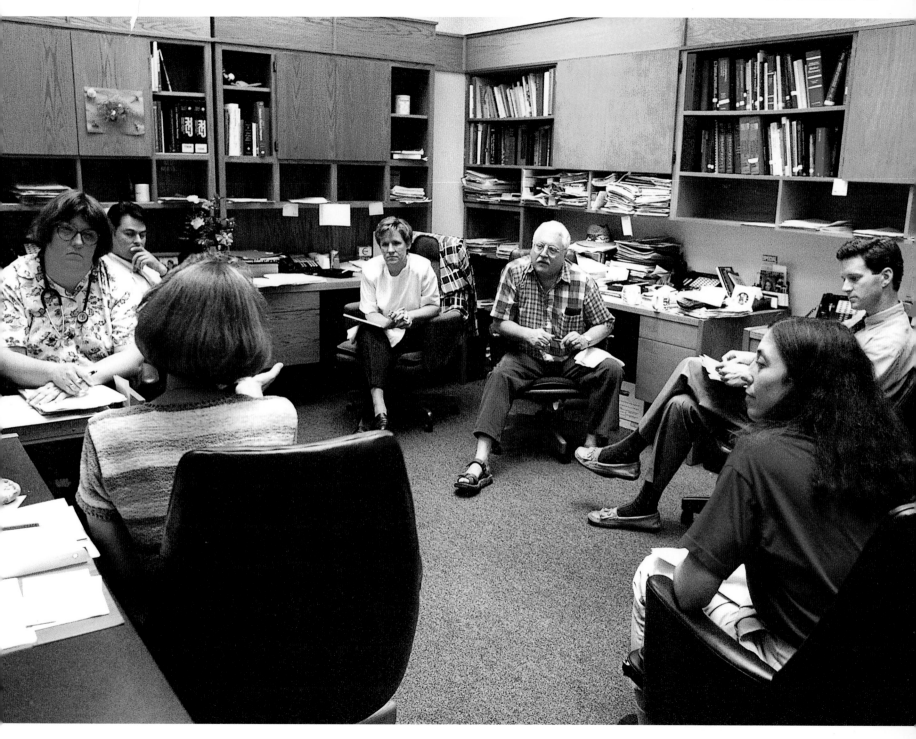

The Clinic Staff

It is so easy for physicians to develop indifference to their clinic staff as they contend with a multitude of ill patients needing help. Doctors may rush from the hospital to the clinic, quickly check messages and hustle into an exam room, neglecting to offer a cheerful good morning to the managers, receptionists, bookkeepers, nurses, assistants and lab techs who make the place function.

For years, Phyllis has reminded her partners that the people of the clinic staff are the front-line ambassadors; they are the first to greet patients as they enter and the last to interact with them as they leave. A good, caring staff is a blessing.

And so the pediatricians spend time planning how they can express appreciation to their employees amidst the hectic pace of clinic that runs from seven a.m. to ten.p.m. daily and has weekend hours. It was decided that special events had to be scheduled where the doctors can interact on a personal basis.

Once a month there is potluck lunch at the clinic with a drawing for such items as movie tickets or free dinners at local restaurants. The people with birthdays are singled out and given flowers with a card signed by all the pediatricians. Everyone has a "secret pal" that gives them gifts on holidays.

All staff members and their families are invited to the annual Christmas dinner and also to the summer picnic. At the softball game that usually precedes the picnic, Phyllis discovered last year that she can still hit the ball hard. But she also found that getting around the bases strains muscles and ligaments that haven't been used since her ball-playing days in college.

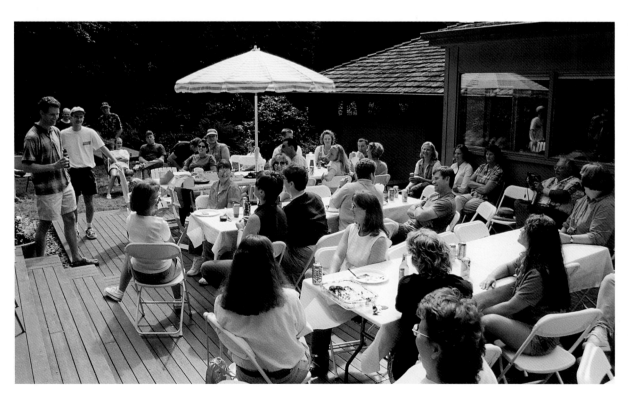

During the 1999 picnic, new pediatricians Randy Copeland and Aidan deRenne share some amusing life experiences, letting the staff know them better.

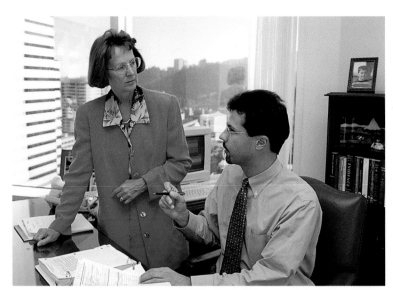

Attorney Jeffrey Street works with Dr. Phyllis Cavens to develop a winning defense in a malpractice suit.

Dealing with the Law

He stands in the clinic hallway, wearing a brown uniform and some sort of official-looking shoulder patch. As the doctor exits from an exam room, their eyes meet in recognition, and they both force a weak smile. The physician is once again greeting "Aggravation," personified in the physical being of the process server.

"Aggravation" hands him a legal document. There is dread as the MD scans the opening words, quickly trying to discover if it is just a summons to give several hours of time testifying for a child in an abuse case or whether it is an announcement that will alter his or her life for several years to come — a notice that the physician is being sued for malpractice.

Though malpractice suits are fairly common, with one in four physicians being eventually hit by one, it is a painful event. Doctors hate the feeling they experience when their competency and dedication are called into question.

... the malpractice suit

Phyllis had hoped that she could retire without facing such a legal struggle, but a child she had saved from immediate death had died many weeks later in a Portland hospital. Months after that, the local hospital, one of her partners and Phyllis were named in a multimillion dollar case.

Whenever doctors face such an ordeal, they find that the slow legal process prolongs the emotional torment. Their malpractice insurance company was fully aware of this and offered them psychological counseling, which they declined.

The insurance company was created by the Washington State Medical Association with the stated purpose of defending against all claims if possible. Over the years, the number of claims in the state of Washington has dropped, since plaintiff attorneys are less likely to sue if the insurance company isn't going to cave in and settle out of court.

The insurance company also hired a lawyer, Jeff Street, to defend it. At their first meeting, Phyllis and her partner were worried that an inexperienced attorney had been pawned off on them, because he looked relatively young. But as Mr. Street carefully outlined the legal troubles they faced, trust in his abilities developed. They in turn taught him the medicine he needed to know.

Together, they brought together six expert witnesses who were quite willing to testify that the care provided was without fault — three pediatricians, a neonatologist, a pediatric gastroenterologist and a pediatric surgeon. The insurance company was paying a lot for defense, but they were determined to win.

... practicing for the deposition

The time had arrived to give depositions. This is a process where both sides sit down to question each other and to determine the strength of each combatant's case. It is a pivotal event, not to be taken lightly, since the recorded testimony can be used months later in a trial, if indeed it proceeds to trial.

Mr. Street invited Phyllis to Portland to practice giving her testimony. His office on the twentieth floor, afforded a panoramic view of the city along the Willamette River. The floors were marble, while the walls were covered in dark cherry wood. Good help did not come cheap.

Mr. Street introduced Phyllis to a smartly-dressed woman, a psychologist who specialized in preparing people for court appearances. As they entered a conference room, Phyllis immediately noticed a mounted video camera. It was placed there to record not only her verbal responses but also her facial expressions and body language.

As the camera rolled, Mr. Street led the nervous pediatrician through those difficult, leading and condescending questions that the plaintiff's attorney was bound to pose. She was taught what she was required to say and how to avoid any legal traps. There was special emphasis on how to handle hypothetical questions. Any question with an **if** posed an assumption of something that hadn't really occurred. "But doctor, what **if** you had...?" "Isn't it true that **if** the diagnosis had...? "Let's assume you..."

The psychologist frequently interrupted Phyllis to criticize her posture, eye contact and gestures. She asserted that the legal process was like a stage play in which Phyllis was acting her small part, with Mr. Street as the director. She even gave instructions on the selection of clothes, makeup, manicure and jewelry, but Phyllis chose to ignore them, not wanting to appear as anything more than a professional doctor.

As they finished, Mr. Street slipped the video tape out of the camera with instructions to Phyllis to review it at home. It had been a disheartening session. But looking at the tape later was even more traumatic. She appeared defensive, like a caged animal, with her voice dropping as she stumbled over uncertain territory.

Her younger partner had gone through the same practice session. A review of that tape revealed an even more shaky performance. This pediatrician, normally so brightly confidant, gave answers that were vague and heart-wrenchingly evasive. The legal process was eating away at that confidence.

Phyllis realized that another practice session was desperately needed, and so she invited her partner to meet at our home. They sat facing each other at the dining room table, taking turns at being an abrasive lawyer.

As the hours went by, it slowly dawned on them that they could handle those tough questions, for they realized that they really had excellent answers. All they had to do was just teach the court the basics of good pediatric practice. They were ready and smiling.

... the deposition

The Cowlitz County Hall of Justice was the scene for Phyllis's deposition. A court reporter was there, along with the parents, the hospital representatives and the doctors. It was the first time all the parties had come face to face. It was an uneasy time.

The deceased child's mother was the first to testify. She acknowledged that her children had always received good care at the clinic and that she liked the doctors. Phyllis began to feel sorry for her when the mother had to reveal details about her personal life. She wondered if the woman now had second thoughts about putting herself through this ordeal and reliving such painful memories.

The opposing attorney, who was a little paunchy and beginning to go bald, started off deceptively low key with his questions. Phyllis was surprised that he allowed her to expand on her personal achievements and on humanitarian efforts with Northwest Medical Teams, an organization that sends medical teams to disasters around the world. But then he quietly began to ask the more pointed questions, and near the last he sprung the dreaded hypotheticals.

PLAINTIFF'S ATTORNEY: *If you had seen that on your first examination, would that have led you ...?*

DR. CAVENS: *You asked me a hypothetical question. What would I do if the appearance of the skin...*

ATTORNEY: *I'm asking you to assume that the operation took place before the ...*

DR. CAVENS: *I will make one comment about the hypothetical and why it's so difficult for a physician to make a response to a hypothetical. Our thought processes are always based on data, and when you take a hypothetical question and throw in something that's improbable, then it's hard for me to process that.*

That didn't stop similar questions. Finally, her lawyer had to object.

MR. STREET: *If you want to ask a hypothetical, lay out the hypothetical. If she can respond she, will. If she can't, she's not required to.*

Her deposition finally ended after four hours. Phyllis felt drained, but as they were walking out of the building, Mr. Street quietly affirmed her performance with a single word of praise: "Perfect."

When she came home, I asked her how it had gone, but she didn't want to make a mental effort to compose her thoughts. She sat down in front of the TV set without eating dinner and stared at some inane program that she really didn't see.

She finally sighed with fatigue, "I just feel like I escaped a car crash."

The Struggle to Stay Independent

One day, Phyllis walked with determination into the kitchen where I was reading the evening paper. She wanted to eat dinner quickly and watch the first televised Portland Trail Blazer basketball game of the shortened season that was starting in just thirty minutes. But there had been two troubling business meetings that day, and her strong desire to see the game was overwhelmed by the need to talk with me about the day's fireworks. The Blazers would have to wait.

There had been an emergency IPA meeting that morning. The IPA, which stands for Independent Practice Association, was a small group of thirty doctors in five clinics struggling not to be swallowed up by big corporations.

The IPA was born three years earlier at the scrub sink. Phyllis and an obstetrician colleague were standing side by side, each using a soap-filled brush to lather first one arm from fingertips to elbow

and then the other. Dressed in scrub greens with only their eyes showing above the surgical masks, it seemed like a clandestine meeting of two spies. And indeed, it was the start of an organized resistance to the forces of corporate medicine.

Phyllis led this small band of private-practice physicians from its inception, but it was very hard. Doctors are by nature independent and often find it difficult to come together, even when that cherished independent status is threatened.

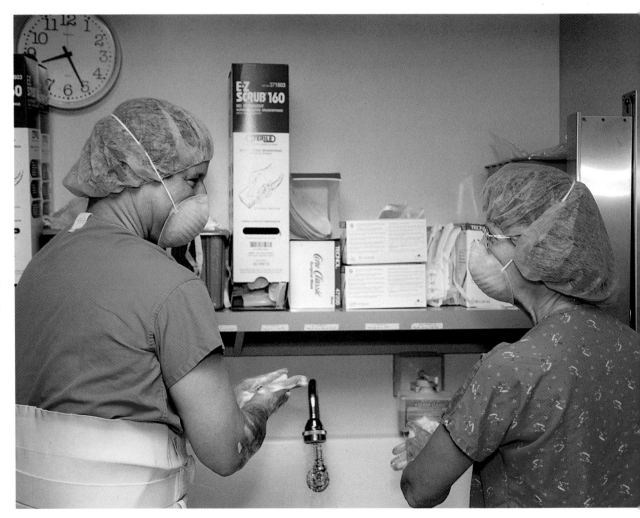

In the same manner as when the IPA started, an obstetrician, Dr. Phillip Henderson, and Phyllis continue planning strategy at the surgical scrub sink.

That day, they learned that one of their five IPA clinics were deserting them to become employees of a "Big Brother." Now, the outside pressures on the IPA were more obvious. A decision had to be made to either give up and dissolve the IPA or move boldly ahead to strengthen it. With her jaw set firmly, Phyllis advised that they hire a part-time administrator to help them continue the struggle. They agreed.

In Bed with HMOs That
Kick the Covers

Though this earlier breakfast meeting with her IPA colleagues had turned out well, the noon meeting with an HMO had been tough. The main item on the agenda had been to settle the coming year's contract. Phyllis and her partners all had rehearsed what they were going to say in hopes of at least getting a cost-of-living increase in their payments.

The HMO had sent several executives in nice suits to do their negotiating. They began by exchanging pleasantries, but then their leader began berating the clinic partners, with an assertion that they were hurting the HMO by not being fully supportive of their goals. The partners remained outwardly calm during the continuing tirade, but inside they were livid with emotion. What was happening? Was the HMO trying to make them react with anger and drop the contract?

Phyllis had coached her partners prior to the meeting that they were to "suck up" to the HMO. And so, Dr. Tolby quietly denied the accusations while Phyllis reasserted that it was not in their clinic's self-interest to denigrate the HMO, but rather to deliver cost-effective, quality care.

The meeting went on for an hour and finally, during the last five minutes, Phyllis was able to bring up the subject of the coming year's fee payments, hoping for at least that cost-of-living increase. An HMO executive asked her what percentage increase she had in mind. She replied that she didn't have a particular number, and countered with, "What are you offering?" Again the HMO rep asked, "What do you want?" And she once more replied, "What can you offer?"

Finally, the HMO made its offer, which was surprisingly quite generous. All the partners sat, startled. They had never expected such an attractive offer, and, in fact, they had been fearful that they were going to be dumped by the HMO. Phyllis calmly replied, "That sounds agreeable. We will get back to you to settle it."

They left the meeting shaken, bewildered once again by their experience with a large insurance company. Why was the firm suddenly so charitable after launching the initial verbal attack? What was their long-term strategy? Phyllis exclaimed later, "I had never felt so much sweat in the armpits of my business suit."

As she recounted that morning's struggle with the IPA and later her encounter with the HMO, I was reminded of a Latin phrase taught us our freshman year in medical school as we faced the coming rigors of medicine — "Non carborundum illigetimi" or "Never let the bastards wear you down."

Though wearied, Phyllis had not been worn down. She was determined to continue with the struggle.

7 ... in the community

Children Need a Medical Home

Phyllis suddenly stiffened in her chair. Her eyes once again read the hospital report to assure her mind that the cold, written words were indeed true.

A 9-month-old baby had been brought to the emergency room and declared dead on arrival. And her name, Dr. Phyllis Cavens, was listed as the baby's personal doctor.

Immediately, a barrage of questions popped forth. "What had happened?" "Why didn't I know?" "Why wasn't I called?" And then the heart-sinking question that all medical people asks themselves whenever there is an unexpected death, "Did I see the child recently and miss some opportunity to prevent this?"

She called for the patient's chart and found the answer to at least one question — an answer that eventually led to a program involving a local charitable foundation, four Rotary clubs, six clinics, the health department and an agency called Parents Place. And it was an answer that led to improved health care for several thousand children.

The dead child had never established a medical home. Dr. Cavens had seen the child only twice during her first week of life, but the little girl had not come back for any further care. There had been no well-baby examinations nor were any immunizations ever given, even though a reminder card had been sent out.

There had been no chance for Phyllis or any of her partners to look for chronic illness, poor growth or neurological impairment. Nor had there been any face-to-face meetings with the mother to teach her how to care for her baby or to look for mental illness in the parent. In addition, no agency or mechanism existed that could have reached down through the cracks to get this child with failing health back into a medical home.

Phyllis was upset. This should not have happened to any patient of hers or any other doctor. She went to Janice Higby, the director of Parents Place, which is a small organization devoted to teaching parents better ways to raise their children. Janice was willing to add a new program if funding could be found for it.

Phyllis suggested that they send a grant proposal to the local Health Care Foundation requesting $42,000 to hire an administrator and staff to track down children who were not immunized. She reasoned that if parents were persuaded to bring their children to a doctor for shots, a medical home would be established and well-child care given.

There was a feeling that the community would back the project. A few years earlier, Longview's St. John Medical Center had conducted a survey and found that only 55 per-

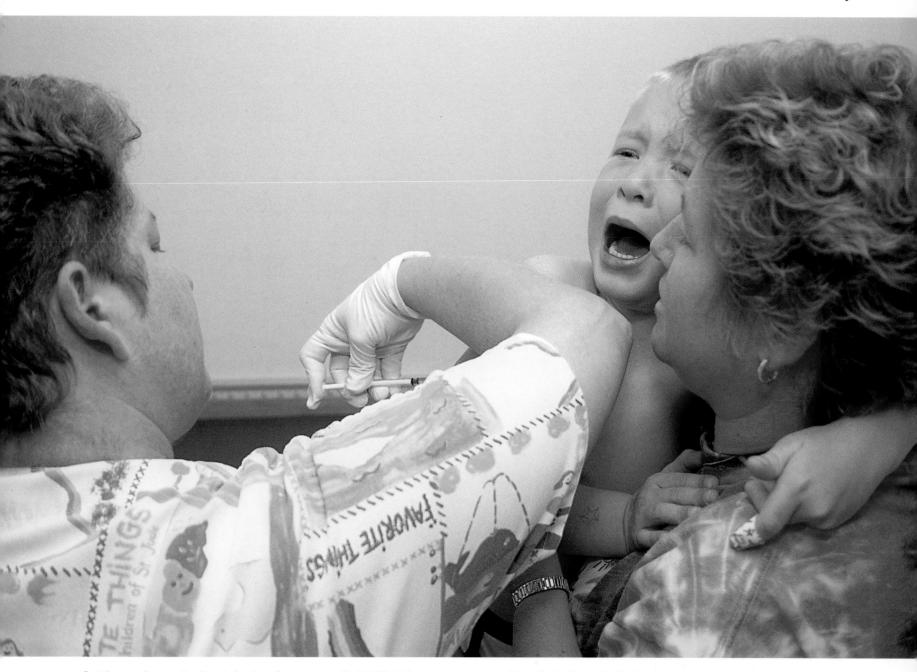

Getting an immunization injection from nurse Debbi Eldridge may not seem friendly to Ryan Dahl, but he does have a medical home at the Child and Adolescent Clinic where his mother, Peggy Dahl, can bring him for comprehensive care. The American Academy of Pediatrics is working to assure that every child in the United States has a similar medical home.

cent of children in the community were fully immunized. In addition, a committee of local leaders, called Pathways 2020, had called for raising the immunization rate to become one of the county's primary health goals.

The grant application was submitted to the Health Care Foundation, but weeks went by without any word. Phyllis was at a social gathering of old friends and began talking to C. C. Bridgewater. Bridgewater is a stocky man. At one time, he could lift more weight than just about any man in Longview, but currently he did his bench work as a judge on the state Court of Appeals. Since he was also on the board of the Health Care Foundation, he knew before she did that the grant had been turned down.

As he informed Phyllis of this, her eyes narrowed and her lips thinned. She pointedly asked why it had failed. The judge smiled slightly and reminded her that the foundation usually gives its money to build "bricks and mortar" projects or to buy sophisticated medical equipment. The pediatrician countered with arguments as to why this project was so important.

Hearing her determination, Bridgewater finally said, "Well, present it again, only this time you go to the meeting of the board and do it personally." She did, and the grant was approved.

At the same time, four local Rotary Clubs were looking for a project that they could work on together. This was it. By pooling their income from various fund-raising activities, they donated $49,000. Parents Place was able, therefore, to expand the program to assist all the doctor groups in the county as they jointly cooperated in tracking down under-immunized

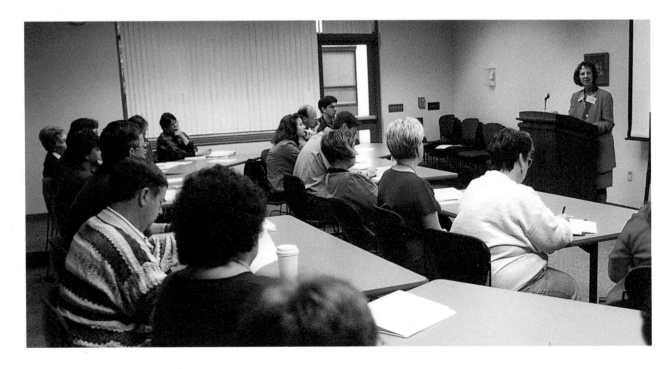

Phyllis participates with leaders of Cowlitz County during a conference on prevention of violence to children. She passed on thoughts of Janet Reno, U.S. Attorney General, and Marion Wright Edelman, founder and president of the Children's Defense Fund, both of whom she heard speak at the 1999 AAP annual meeting.

children in the entire area.

In a year's time, the immunization rate rose from the dismal 55 percent to over 88 percent but, more importantly, many more children found a medical home where they would have access to 24-hour care by their doctors on an ongoing, personal basis. The chances of another child dying because of neglect or missed disease had been vastly reduced.

Partnering in the Community

An offhand remark made by ABC co-anchor Charles Gibson while covering the trial of an 11-year-old boy accused of murder was understandable. He had sighed: "What can we do to *protect ourselves* against such children?" But Phyllis was appalled. She felt that question should have been, "What can we do to *protect children* against the abuse and neglect that leads them to erupt in horrible violence?"

That was a turning point for her. Earlier, Janice Higby, the director of Parents Place, had asked Phyllis to participate in a community conference called "Cowlitz Cares," devoted to protection of children from violence, but she had declined. But that was back then, before Charlie Gibson's comment. With new determination, she gathered information and the thoughts of national leaders about violence prevention while attending the American Academy of Pediatrics 1999 annual meeting in Washington, D.C. Phyllis returned to Longview to be part of the "Cowlitz Cares" conference, meeting with the leaders of the community agencies who also worried about the welfare of children. Together they partnered.

"Partnering" is a key word if effective community programs are going to be developed for children. The AAP has recognized the value that a pediatrician brings to any such effort and awards grants under a program called CATCH. The grants are meant to support the planning of worthwhile community projects.

There are other forms of partnering that are necessary if new medical services are to be brought to children. One such

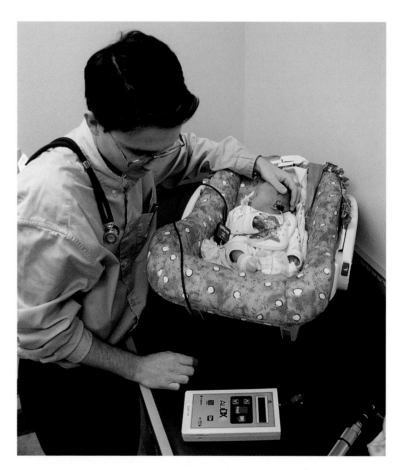

Dr. Aidan deRenne tests four-day-old Alec Sadle with an OAE instrument, a $4000 electronic device used to screen newborns for hearing loss, a new medical service.

new service is the examination of newborns for normal hearing. There is conclusive proof now that if a deaf baby does not hear sound at a very early age, nerve pathways will never connect that later in life might make hearing aids useful. On the other hand, if hearing loss in a newborn is found immediately, hearing aids can be provided, giving the baby a much greater chance of developing good speech.

Pediatrician Dr. Aidan deRenne worked with the staff of St. John Medical Center to create a special program for screening all new babies for normal hearing. He was able to provide the expensive equipment and the trained staff to quickly set up the service so that babies with impaired hearing would not be missed.

Helping the Nation's Children

As Phyllis and I exited a taxi in Washington, D.C., we gazed skyward in awe at the Cannon Building. I continued to look up once inside the office of U.S. Rep. Pete Stark. The height of the ceiling was probably three times the width of the small waiting room we were in. This was a disappointment, because I would not be able to bounce my camera flash off the ceiling to get a natural-looking photograph of Congressman Stark and Dr. Joel Alpert.

Dr. Alpert was meeting with the congressman to personally acquaint him with a new proposal from the American Academy of Pediatrics to provide health insurance for all children of the United States. As president of the AAP, he had delivered a speech two days earlier unveiling the proposal to thousands of pediatricians at their annual convention. They had risen to their feet with grateful emotion to applaud his efforts.

The height of the room seemed somehow appropriate when Pete Stark entered to fill the door frame. He was tall and angular with a gentle smile that softened his craggy face. He graciously pulled two chairs in front of his desk so that I could take pictures using light from the outside window.

The two men sat down to face each other while their young staffers, seated several feet away, leaned forward with intensity to hear the ensuing conversation. These were men of prestige and power. Dr. Alpert was a professor of pediatrics and public health at Boston City Hospital; Rep. Stark from Califronia was a senior member of the Ways and Means Committee and a ranking member of the Health Subcommittee. Both were champions of universal health insurance.

Dr. Alpert presented the congressman a blue-colored sheet outlining the proposal. Stark listened carefully and remarked on one point, "That's not hard." He asked some questions that Alpert answered and offered suggestions. It dawned on me that these gentlemen — and I use the term in its original intent — *gentle men* — were developing a strategy that might indeed help millions of children.

I marveled at how the two seemed so at ease with each other; there seemed to be a genuine friendship. A clue to their relationship revealed itself just as we were preparing to leave. The scene suddenly changed as Congressman Stark pulled his chair close to Dr. Alpert and began talking in lowered tones that left the rest of us out of the conversation.

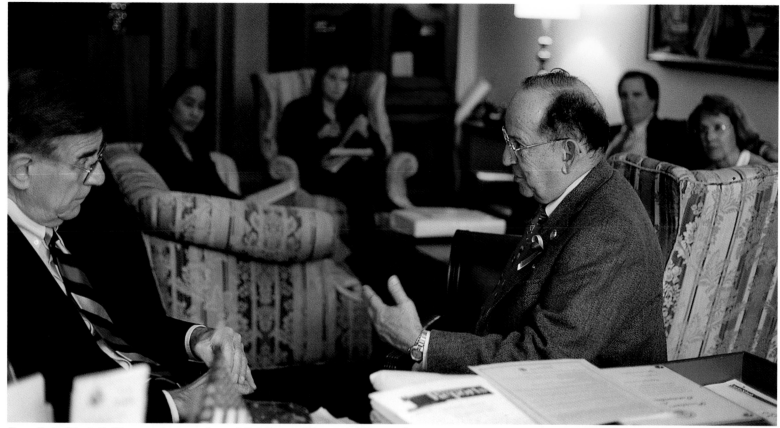

Rep. Pete Stark (left), a senior member of the House Ways and Means Committee, listens intently to Dr. Joel Alpert who, as President of the American Academy of Pediatrics, helped develop the organization's proposal for the United States to provide health insurance for all its children.

I looked back over my shoulder to see that he was showing pictures to the doctor. It was obvious that these were not photos of fishing trips or golf courses that men of success might exhibit, but rather they were of a child. I glanced around the room to see that there were other pictures of children posing with family members. There were so many photos that cluttered the top of a nearby desk that one framed enlargement of a child was relegated to placement on the floor. This then was part of the rapport between the congressman and the pediatrician — a mutual love of children.

Dr. Alpert continued to chuckle approval as Rep. Stark flipped through the photos of the child. It occurred to me that this one child might be a link in a matrix of events that would eventually help 11 million uninsured children.

"There is only one child in the world; and the child's name is all children." — Carl Sandburg

Helping the World

Because of their training and experience, pediatricians have a unique opportunity to help in world disasters such as famine, flood, or war. In such situations, children are the most vulnerable segment of the afflicted population; consequently, when help finally arrives, they are often found dying of starvation, pneumonia, dehydration or septic shock. The pediatrician discovers that his or her specialized skills — skills that may be used in emergencies back home once or twice a month to save a child from the brink of death — are often needed in disaster situations many times a day. It is very soul satisfying.

Phyllis has been learning that lesson since 1979, when she joined the first group that Northwest Medical Teams sent to Thailand to treat the Cambodian refugees, victims of the "killing fields." Since then, she has been to Ethiopia, Somalia, Mexico, Jamaica, Uzbekistan, and Honduras, where she and her teammates have been able to reach out and help people.

... Ethiopia — "We are the World"

In 1985, a disastrous famine hit Ethiopia and the world turned its attention to the tragedy with the biggest outpouring of aid that had ever been seen. That time is often remembered by the song, "We Are the World," written by Michael Jackson and Quincy Jones and recorded by 45 famous singers and other celebrities who came together to raise funds.

Dr. Phyllis flew on a World Vision twin-prop plane to Ibnat,

The Song and the Singers

"We are the World.
We are the people.
We are the ones who
 make a brighter day,
 so let's start giving."

Dan Aykroyd-Harry Belafonte-Lindsey Buckingham-Kim Carnes-Ray Charles-Bob Dylan-Sheila E.-Bob Geldof-Daryl Hall & John Oates-James Ingram-Jackie Jackson-La Toya Jackson-Marlon Jackson-Michael Jackson-Randy Jackson-Tito Jackson-Al Jarreau-Waylon Jennings-Billy Joel-Cyndi Lauper-Huey Lewis & The News-Kenny Loggins-Bette Midler-Willie Nelson-Jeffrey Osborne-Steve Perry-The Pointer Sisters-Lionel Richie-Smokey Robinson-Kenny Rogers-Dianna Ross-Paul Simon-Bruce Springsteen-Tina Turner-Dionne Warwick-Stevie Wonder

---

the site of a refugee camp high in the mountains of Ethiopia. Cholera struck the camp a few days after her team arrived.

Cholera is a very serious disease. About 70 percent of patients who get it die of shock, since watery diarrhea pours forth unabated. On the other hand, it is an exciting and satisfying disease for doctors to treat. Most patients will recover in three days if enough fluid is poured in by mouth or IV to match the fluid coming out.

At Ibnat, people with cholera covered the floor of their medical tent, a tent that could only hold 200 patients. Since there were no beds, doctors and nurses crouched on the floor to start IVs, sometimes with the aid of a flashlight in the night darkness. As patients recovered, more would take their place.

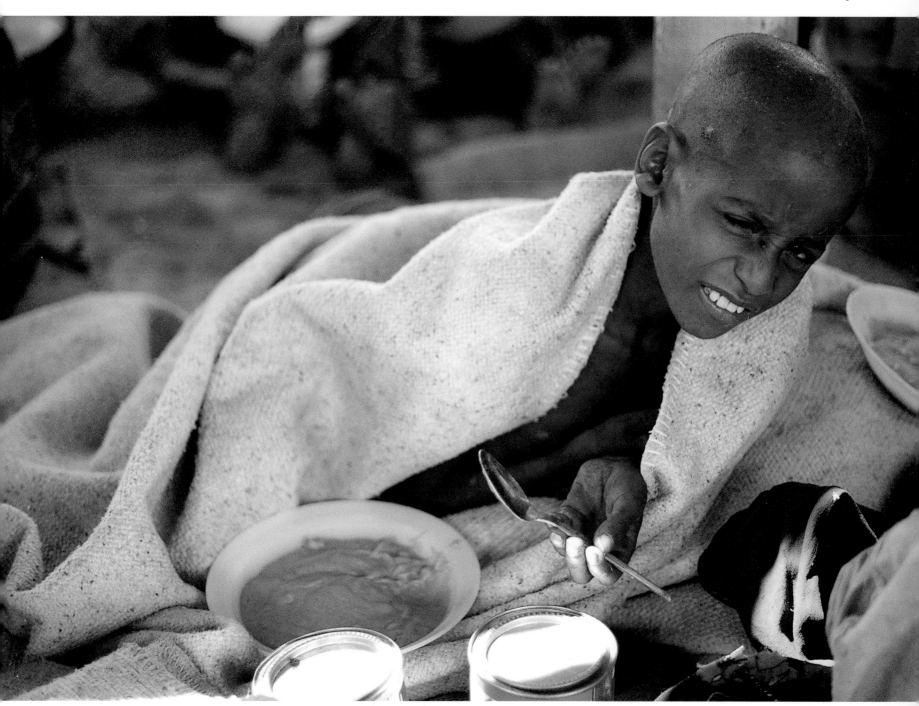

An Ethiopian boy, victim of the 1985 famine, struggles to eat the emergency rations prepared for him by an international aid agency.

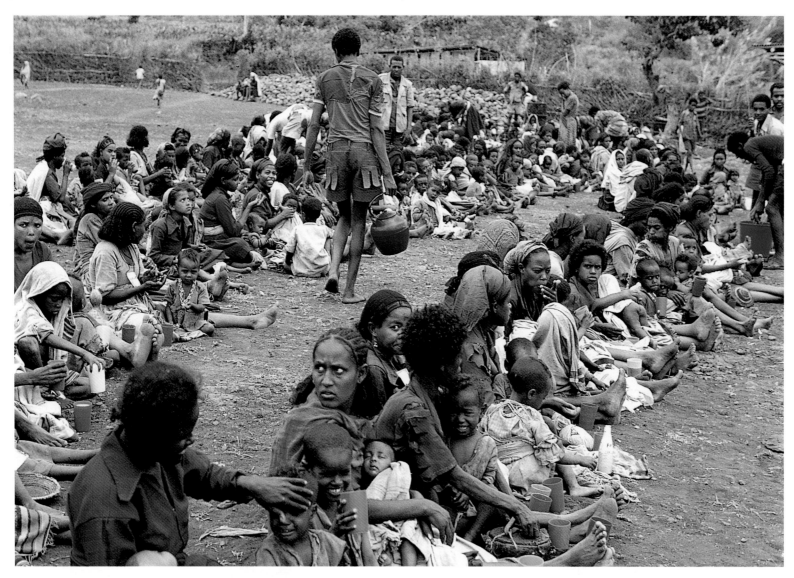

Above: Mothers wait for milk for their children to be distributed during the 1985 Ethiopian famine. A population was saved through international efforts.

Far right: Dr. Phyllis Cavens directs help for this starving Somali child during the 1992 crisis. She led a group of doctors and nurses from Northwest Medical Teams. Team photo

When the epidemic finally waned after a week, 600 people had been treated, but only 6 had died. If the team had not been there, more than 400 would have succumbed. Ron Post, the founder of Northwest Medical Teams, reflected that the effort was equivalent to saving all the people on the jumbo jet he flew home on.

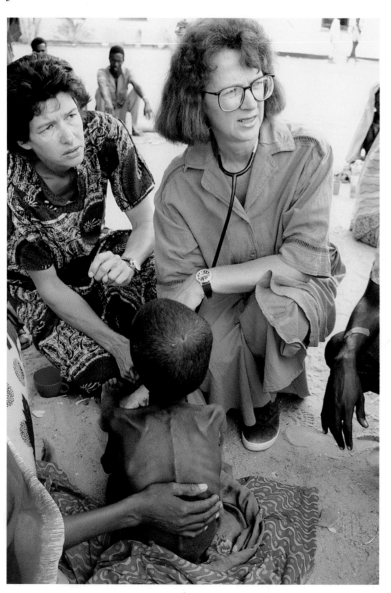

... Somalia

Twin terrors hit Somalia in 1992: war and famine. While the United States sent in the Marines to assist, Northwest Medical Teams provided successive groups of medical personnel. As is so often the case in overseas work, these doctors and nurses faced not only disease and starvation, but also the impact of major cultural differences. Phyllis personally experienced how cruelly women can be treated in some countries.

When the medical team traveled to one of the village huts, Phyllis discovered a woman and her two small children who were too ill to get up and walk. She saw a group of men standing close by and through her interpreter asked two of them to carry the little ones to the clinic. Immediately, laughter broke out among all the men.

Bewildered, she turned to her interpreter to find out what was so funny. As he continued laughing along with the men, he responded that men don't carry children, and, more importantly, a woman never orders a man in that country to perform a task. So Phyllis gathered the children in her own arms and carried them

One day, a young Somali woman was brought to the local hospital. Her genitalia had been slashed with a machete during a raid by a rival tribe that had killed the men and mutilated the women. The girl was taken to the operating room, which had open windows because it was so hot. A nurse was given the task of chasing the flies away from the surgical field.

As the reparative surgery was being done, the surgeon showed Phyllis results of the patient's prior female circumcision. The inner labia had been removed and the vaginal opening had been sewn shut. (A few days later, the operative wound was healing well without getting infected.)

When the team first arrived at the Kenya-Somali border, they met the administrator who had been hired to be the ground coordinator for the team. His job was to provide them with the basics of living and transportation. But he was incompetent and often ignored their needs, traveling off with his driver on various personal errands.

One morning as he was leaving, Phyllis furiously ran out to the truck and shouted at him to provide them with the breakfast he had neglected to get. There was further argument until he agreed to get them food. She learned years later that, as his truck sped out of the compound that day, raising red dust, his driver turned to him and said, "Do you want me to have her killed?"

... Honduras

Treating the victims of Hurricane Mitch was a different experience. More than three feet of rain had fallen in a few hours one night in late October, 1998, tearing out buildings, roads, and bridges. It also contaminated the water.

Phyllis and four other members of Northwest Medical Teams flew to the mountains of Northern

Honduras to help the villagers that had been isolated by the high water and washed-out roads. Many of the children had developed abscesses on their legs after walking in sewer-filled mud. Others suffered from bloody diarrhea due to drinking infected water.

A 16-day-old baby, born during the hurricane in filthy conditions, was in septic shock when she was brought to the doctors. By giving the little girl IV fluids and antibiotics, they were able to save her life.

Their medical efforts took a different direction, however,

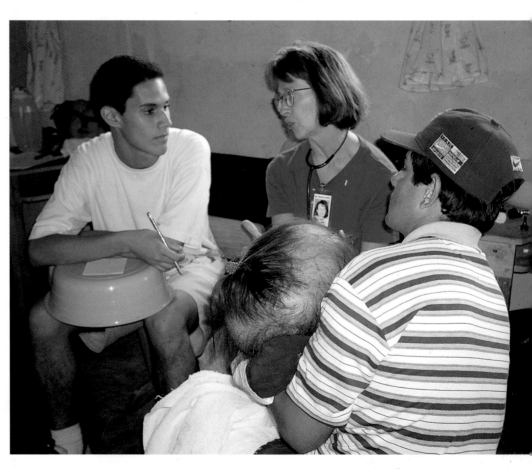

Honduran Children Discovered by Team and Sent for Specialty Care

18-month-old boy with hydrocephalus with a shunt, but no recent care.

15-year-old boy with bed wetting and leg weakness — a possible tethered spinal cord.

15-month-old girl with untreated seizures.

7-year-old boy with a stricture of the penile urethra.

10-year-old blind boy with microcephaly.

10-month-old boy with a white pupil — probable retinoblastoma, a cancer starting in the eye.

2-year-old boy with left facial and leg weakness — probable brain tumor.

11-month-old boy with decreased vision after typhoid fever.

10-year-old boy with spastic quadriplegia — needing a wheelchair.

7-year-old girl with a dislocated knee causing a flail leg.

5-year-old boy with spastic quadriplegia after meningitis.

4-year-old girl with a peri-rectal abscess.

9-month-old blind girl.

3-year-old boy with a left club foot.

9-month-old girl with a heart murmur — and possible trisomy 15 or 18.

2-year-old boy failing to grow and with clubbing of his fingers — possible cystic fibrosis.

8-month-old with a loud heart murmur — undiagnosed congenital heart disease.

2-year-old with probable coarctation of the aorta.

---

when a father came to their makeshift clinic, carrying what appeared to be a large pillow in his arms. On closer look, Phyllis realized that the "pillow" was really a child's head dilated to four times its normal size by "water on the brain," or hydrocephalus. In addition, the little 19-month-old girl was blind and could not move her legs. Yet this father loved her and had protected her during the hurricane. He was now bringing his child to them for some hope.

Phyllis introduced herself and, as she talked, she stroked the child's hand. She was startled when the little fingers suddenly gripped her own and the girl said, "Hello, doctor."

The child's name was Mercy. Phyllis felt some effort had to be made to help Mercy. Through Padre Andreas, they contacted the Sisters of Caretas to see if they would facilitate getting Mercy to a major medical center if Northwest Medical Teams provided funds for transportation and housing. The sisters agreed.

Far left: Allan Zelaya listens to directions from Phyllis in order to translate them to the father of Mercy, who cradles her huge head in his left arm.

Team photo

That meeting with Mercy changed the focus of the team. Having taken care of most of the acute illnesses, they began looking for children with chronic disease conditions in an effort to get them the help they had never had up in the mountains of this poor country. In two weeks, they found case after case of conditions that pediatricians in the United States see only occasionally.

The team made arrangements with Caretas for all these children to go to Tegucigalpa, the capital, for specialty care; an effort started because a caring father brought to them his Mercy, so that they could, in return, practice mercy.

How different this father was from the men of Somalia.

As the team was finally leaving to go back to the U.S., their young Honduran translator gave Phyllis a letter in which he wrote, "How can I begin to thank you for the Honduran people and myself in particular. There are just no words ... Your time here, though it might seem short, will last a lifetime. I will make sure of it."

"With love. Allan Zelaya"

8 ... and the rewards

Pediatrics is a demanding profession with its stresses of treating very ill children, making hospital rounds and being on call. But there are abundant rewards.

There is, of course, a good income, which varies with the location in the United States and the practice situation. In 1998, a work year shortened by her spending three weeks in Honduras, Phyllis earned $156,836. In addition, $29,956 was set aside for her in a retirement program. She drives a 1995 Toyota Land Cruiser, her children are through college, and the mortgage on the house in the woods is retired. Blessed with good health, she and the family have had adventurous vacations throughout the world

But thirty years of practice has brought more than physical comforts. There is no greater satisfaction than being called "doctor" and being known as a caring healer. If a pediatrician has been in practice any length of time, he or she will certainly encounter a man or woman who approaches them on the street and says, "Do you remember, Doctor, the time you saved my child's life?" And often the pediatrician is embarrassed because he or she truly can't remember specifically, because there have been so many patients through the years. But to that parent, it was the major event in their lives.

Or patients who have grown

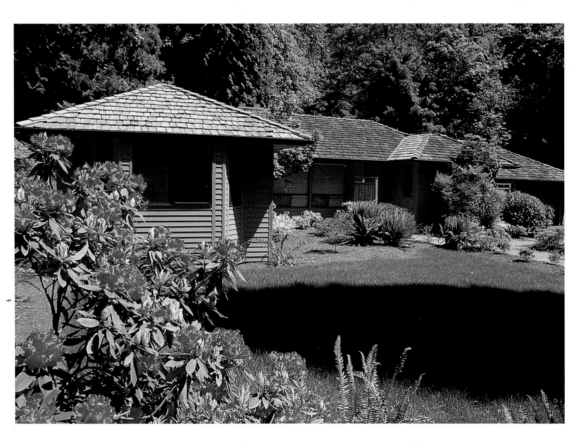

Rhododendrons bloom at the Cavens' home in Washington state.

into adults will encounter the pediatrician and reminisce about a very difficult time in their life. Phyllis recently was thrilled to talk to two of her former patients.

... Sarah

Sarah Manchester was only five years old when her parents brought her to see Phyllis and leukemia was discovered. That was seventeen years ago. Recently, when I called her mother, Marilyn Manchester, to ask if Sarah was coming home for Christmas and if she might agree to have her story told, I felt some remorse. Marilyn said that they hadn't thought about Sarah's ordeal for years, and I realized belatedly that I might be bringing up painful memories.

But Sarah did call at Christmas and came to the clinic along with her husband, Colby Phillips, in addition to her mother and her father, Mike Manchester. It turned out to be a happy reunion, with Phyllis bubbling with excitement as they recounted what part she had in saving this now grown woman from death.

At the start, little kindergartner Sarah had been suffering with arm and chest pain, decreased appetite, tiredness and spasms of coughing. She had been given several rounds of antibiotics without results at another clinic, where it was suggested that she see a psychiatrist to sort out "emotional" symptoms. Her parents were both worried and frustrated as they came to see Dr. Phyllis Cavens for the first time.

The Manchesters remembered well that after examining Sarah, Phyllis had said that there was indeed something seriously wrong with Sarah and that they were going to find out what. She felt a swelling in Sarah's neck and arranged for a biopsy. Later, when she disclosed that the test results showed an ominous cancer, the Manchesters experienced a strange but very common reaction: They were relieved. Now they had the name of a disease. Now they knew what they were up against and could prepare to fight it.

At Children's Hospital in Seattle, they were plunged into a world of rapid learning. They discovered that there were many forms of cancer, and that Sarah had ALL, or acute lymphocytic leukemia, which gave her only a fifty-fifty chance of survival.

They learned about the different cells in the blood and how potent drugs affected each kind. They were given eleven pages of instructions on how to give medicines at home through a Hickman line, a thin tube that was surgically planted in Sarah's small chest and rested inside her heart.

Sarah began chemotherapy with repeating cycles of drugs that would go on for nearly three years. Each cycle was 23 weeks long and would start with her at Children's Hospital for four days to receive extremely high doses of cancer fighting medicines. She would then go home, and for the next 22 weeks she would get many of her medicines from her parents who had very specific directions to follow.

The instructions varied each week. For instance, during Week 6 they were to give methotrexate twice during that time and 6MP four times. When Week 7 came, Mom or Dad would administer an IV dose of vincristine through her implanted

IV catheter (Hickman line) and give her prednisone by mouth. They would take her to the clinic for an injection of L-Aspariginase into her leg. Week 8 was to be a repeat of Week 7, but as Week 9 started, the medicines would change again. There were five doses of cyclophosamide to remember to give. And so the barrage of medicines continued for a total of 22 weeks, until it was time to go to Children's Hospital and start another 23-week cycle all over again.

There were multiple visits to Phyllis and countless samples of blood drawn to check the effects of the drugs. In addition, Sarah had to endure spinal taps and the painful procedure of blood being sucked out of her bone marrow for analysis.

Many problems arose, such as repeated plugging of her implanted Hickman intravenous line — her lifeline. Sarah's blood counts were a constant worry also, since if they fell too low as a reaction to her cancer drugs, she would be unable to fight off common germs that could kill her.

And now as the participants were looking back on this history, other memories, etched permanently by emotional stress, were resurrected. Sarah's father, Mike, remembered a little girl who bit his finger as he tried to get her to swallow medicine, but Phyllis had achieved compliance by quietly saying with strong determination, "You have to do this. I am going to win here, Sarah."

Mike Manchester, a man who speaks with a soft smile, also recalled how his heart sagged when he and this spunky little girl of five were walking on the farm and she said to him, "I am very lucky. Either I take my medicine and lick this, or I die and go to heaven."

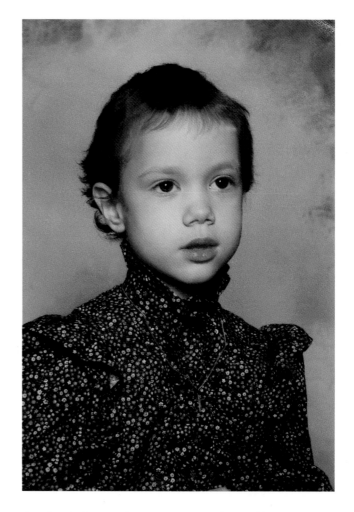

A school picture shows 5-year-old Sarah Manchester at the time she was being treated for leukemia.

Family photo

She had taken her medicine, starting seventeen years ago, and that afternoon stood before the group as a beautiful, vibrant woman preparing for a career in nursing. All were joyous including her new husband, her loving parents, and, of course, Dr. Phyllis, who once again was privileged to feel the warmth of playing a part in the saving of a life.

Sarah with her husband, Colby Phillips, visit Phyllis during the Christmas season and review the scrapbook that her mother had kept during the fight against leukemia — so successfully won.

... Billy

Dr. Phyllis Cavens was absorbed as she leafed through Billy Smith's chart. Billy was coming to meet her and have his picture taken for this book; however, he was no longer Billy, but 20-year-old Bill.

The chart was more than an inch and a half thick, typical for a child with a chronic illness and frequent visits. Inside its worn cover were packets of decade-old lab reports and transcriptions, plus page after page of scribbled notes.

As Phyllis read those notes, she recalled the many anxious moments during that year-and-a-half struggle to conquer this little boy's bone cancer in his leg. It wasn't, however, the written word that caused the strongest emotional response within her, but rather a picture.

Stapled to the inside of the chart cover were a series of Christmas card photos of Billy with his brother. Both boys are happy and smiling in all of them, except for the one in which Billy is seen sitting in an oversized chair while his brother stands. Though he is smartly dressed in a suit, the affects of his chemotherapy are obvious. A stylishly matching cap on his head hides his baldness, but it doesn't cover a wasted face that is trying valiantly to muster a smile.

Phyllis had just closed his chart and made a soulful remark about how ghastly he looked in the old picture when word arrived that Billy, or rather Bill, was in the waiting room. We both went to greet him and found a charming young man

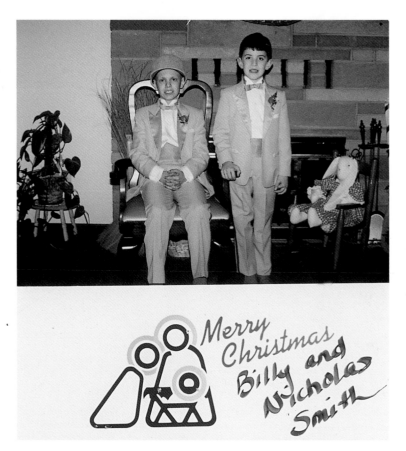

An ill Billy Smith poses with his brother, Nicholas, for the Christmas card that was sent to Dr. Cavens at the time.

Family photo

whose handsome smile drew us to him immediately.

His attitude was so mature. He listened intently to our words, unlike so many youth who dismiss their elders as irrelevant. It made me think of a monologue by humorist Garrison Keillor in which he muses that young people are often so full of themselves until that time when they experience some harsh reality. Bill, unlike most adolescents, had faced pain and death many times before even reaching age eleven. He had learned the value of supportive relationships and kind-

Dr. Cavens visits Bill Smith at the University of Washington campus in Seattle, where he is finishing his sophomore year's study in chemical engineering.

ness at a much earlier point in his life.

And now he was a sophomore at the University of Washington, studying chemical engineering. During the summers, he worked at the local Weyerhauser Company paper mill to earn the money for his schooling. He loved to water and snow ski.

But it might not have been so. When he was nine, he developed Ewing's sarcoma, a cancer that was destroying the bone in his left knee. It is a disease that used to kill 85 percent of the patients.

But little Billy had lots of help in successfully fighting it. There were the doctors and nurses at Children's Hospital in Seattle who started him on chemotherapy and radiation treatment. He recalls walking around half asleep on IV medications. In spite of the seriousness of his condition he was surprised as to how jolly his doctors were. It helped him in adjusting to the inevitable chaos of hospital life.

His mother always stayed with him in the hospital and made friends with the other children and parents to the point that they all began to feel like family. But it was a family in which there were inevitable tragedies. Bill remembered that one of his good friends finally died of leukemia.

In between stays in Seattle, Dr. Phyllis provided his cancer care. The toughest problem was that his IV medicines made him vomit, but he had to have them on a regular basis. He wouldn't sleep well for several nights prior to the coming round of medicine. Dr. Phyllis ordered alternating doses of Benadryl, Reglan and Lorazepam every two hours before and after the cancer drugs were given intravenously, trying desperately to relieve the little boy's retching.

To make life easier when this weak, bald child first returned to school, the principal, JoAnn Robinson, arranged to have Phyllis come and explain the disease to his classmates.

By age eleven, Billy had whipped the cancer, and there was a celebration party for him at the clinic as they declared him well. Bill remembers that his nurse from Seattle came down for the celebration. But she was just one of many who had invested themselves in his survival. Besides his family, there were lab technicians, nurses, cancer specialists and his primary care physician, Dr. Phyllis Cavens.

Our visit with an adult Bill came to a close admidst the happy conversation of saying goodbye. But Bill interrupted the laughter with a solemn declaration. He looked directly into the eyes of Phyllis to be sure that she heard him and that she understood his feeling, and quietly declared, "I wouldn't be here if it weren't for you."

Being an Inspiration

In the Greek classic, the Odyssey by Homer, the goddess Athena speaks words of encouragement to the son of Ulysses: "I look with hope on your undertaking." She does this, however, disguised as the old family friend, Mentor -- hence our modern term, mentoring.

Mentoring is not an act of giving direct advice, but rather, it is one of listening, encouraging and being an inspiration. All pediatricians are mentors. They represent to young ones the compassionate side of humanity to counterbalance the multitude of Rambo-like images.

Often doctors are unaware of the influence they have over individual children. Even little things, such as the selection of the office decor can change a child's life.

... Jessica

This was expressed in a letter Phyllis recently received from Margaret Barton-Ross, a mother who had recently visited her grown daughter, Jessica, who was serving in the Peace Corps in South Africa. She wrote, "We were talking about the various things that sparked her interest in Africa. One of the big influences in her young life was you ... But also amusingly enough, she was taken as a child by the decor of your examining rooms. Those photographs and batiks of the animals of Africa caught her imagination."

And so the seemingly insignificant pictures on the wall of animals photographed while Phyllis and her family were on safari had been a subtle turning point in the life of this young woman.

A little girl, Mosebjane Koktelo, sits atop the shoulders of Jessica Ross, a Peace Corps worker in South Africa. Jessica's interest in Africa was stimulated by the pictures of animals on the walls of the Child and Adolescent Clinic that had been taken while Phyllis was on safari with her family.
Family photo

... Jeff

Pediatricians can be mentors more directly. In 1992, a college student, Jeff Flaskerud, accompanied Phyllis and a youth team from Emmanuel Lutheran Church in Longview on a short-term mission project to Arizona. Since he had an interest in going to medical school, he worked with her as

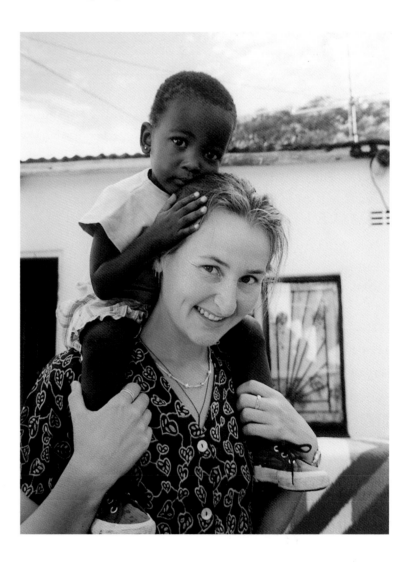

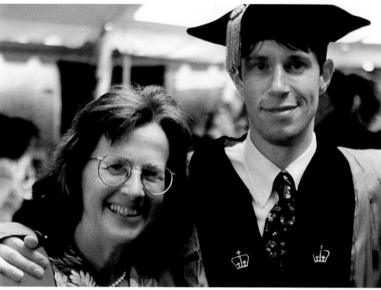

Dr. Jeff Flaskerud gives a hug to his inspiration, Dr. Phyllis Cavens,
at the time of his graduation from medical school.

Family photo

she donated time at the Navajo Nation's hospital in Chinle.

He told her back then that if he ever did get into medical school and graduate, he would invite her to the ceremony. She was pleased that he had such a dream and promised she would attend if he did. When he was home for Christmas six years later, he proudly informed her of his impending graduation from Columbia University Medical School and reminded her of the promise. Even though the ceremony was to be clear across the United States, she flew there that following May.

All the new doctors opened their diplomas at graduation to find tucked inside the original essay they each had composed years earlier in applying to Columbia. Jeff had written, "I have a friend, Phyllis Cavens, who is a pediatrician.

Phyllis is a member of Northwest Medical Teams, and she has gone with the teams to the aid of many third world countries. I have listened to some of her stories, and I would find satisfaction in bringing aid to people as she does. She is one of my heroes."

Soon after receiving his MD degree that day, Jeff began a pediatric residency program so that in three years he would begin his career of

... being a pediatrician.

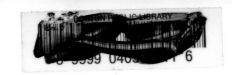